THE BEAUTY IN BREAKING

THE
BEAUTY
IN
BREAKING

A MEMOIR

Michele Harper

RIVERHEAD BOOKS
NEW YORK
2020

RIVERHEAD BOOKS
An imprint of Penguin Random House LLC

Copyright © 2020 by Michele Harper
Penguin supports copyright. Copyright fuels creativity, encourages diverse
voices, promotes free speech, and creates a vibrant culture. Thank you for
buying an authorized edition of this book and for complying with copyright
laws by not reproducing, scanning, or distributing any part of it in any form
without permission. You are supporting writers and allowing Penguin
to continue to publish books for every reader.

Riverhead and the R colophon are registered trademarks of
Penguin Random House LLC.

ISBN 9780525537380

Printed in the United States of America

Book design by Amanda Dewey

AUTHOR'S NOTE

I have intentionally altered some details in this manuscript, particularly identifying details concerning patients, colleagues, various hospitals, and other locations. While names and dates may have been changed, the human experience at the center of this story is true and unfolded as described.

To the truth tellers and the truth seekers;
to those who live honestly now and to the others
who will one day; and last, but not least,
to those courageous enough to love in a way
that only creates freedom

CONTENTS

Introduction   xi

ONE. *Michele: A Wing and a Prayer*   1

TWO. *Dr. Harper: The View from Here*   21

THREE. *Baby Doe: Born Perfect*   45

FOUR. *Erik: Violent Behavior Alert*   70

FIVE. *Dominic: Body of Evidence*   93

SIX. *Jeremiah: Cradle and All*   113

SEVEN. *In the Name of Honor*   138

EIGHT. *Joshua: Under Contract*   166

NINE. *Paul: Murda, Murda*   204

TEN. *Sitting with Olivia*   234

ELEVEN. *Jenny and Mary: What Falls Away*   257

Epilogue   278

ACKNOWLEDGMENTS   281
WORKS CITED   283

INTRODUCTION

*God breaks the heart again and again
and again until it stays open.*

—HAZRAT INAYAT KHAN

As I CRADLED MY patient's head in my hands, I looked past the watery wells of his eyes. For a moment, I didn't notice the blood that ran in rivulets across my gloves as it poured from his scalp, or the bits of gray and white brain matter that dotted the sheets. The beeping of the monitors around me, the popping sound of IV catheter tops being flicked off by nurses, the screeching of wheels as equipment was dragged across linoleum floors, the nurses and techs yelling directions at one another, the stifled gasps erupting from the two medical students on their first ER shift attempting in vain not to be startled—all were drowned out as I stood over this young man and tried to ease his agitation.

This is the part of being a doctor that medical school doesn't cover, that case reviews don't prepare you for. This is the part you can't really know until you're in the moment: You are the person responsible for saving the human life that slowly slips through your fingers while silently begging for final redemption under the demanding fluorescent lights.

I am the doctor whose palms bolster the head of the twenty-year-old man with a gunshot wound to his brain. I support the baby as she takes her first breath outside her mother's womb. I hug the wife whose husband is dying from advanced liver disease as she implores the universe to take away his pain.

I claim no special powers; nor do I know how to handle death any better than you. What I know is that for thirty-six hours a week, I reside in the melee that is a hospital emergency room, where I am called upon to be salve, antidote, and sometimes Charon. Most of the time my job is to keep death at bay. When I am successful, I send the patient back out into the world. When I'm not, I am there as life passes away.

I'm not so deluded as to think that I alone am capable of making that kind of difference. I'm well aware that the determination of who lives and who dies doesn't happen at my hands alone. There are times when, despite the designs of any patient, family member, friend, or doctor, death will come. Then I am witness. What I can do is be the ferry-woman who holds the body as the last breath escapes, the one who, like the night sentinel, calls out the hour and does her best to convey that all is well.

Like everyone, I am in this world for only a brief time. And as for many, blessings abound in my life, and they abound amid the struggle, amid *my* struggle. Over the decades I've learned to cultivate a personal state of stillness. As a child, that stillness grew from a dissociation I stumbled upon that allowed me to better endure life with a father who was a batterer and with a family legacy of victimhood. As a black woman, I navigate an American landscape that claims to be post-racial when every waking moment reveals the contrary, an American landscape that requires all women to pound tenaciously against the proverbial glass ceiling, which we've since discovered is made of palladium, the kind of glass that would sooner bow than shatter.

When I began writing this book, I had started over. My marriage to my college sweetheart had ended. I had moved to a new city to start a new job. Plagued with doubt, I found myself having to reevaluate my life. Living through such changes was difficult; now I see those junctures, when everything I had counted on came to an abrupt end, as a privilege. They gave me the opportunity to be uncertain. And in that uncertainty grew opportunity.

From childhood to now, I have been broken many times. I suspect most people have. In practicing the Japanese art of Kintsukuroi, one repairs broken pottery by filling in the cracks with gold, silver, or platinum. The choice to highlight the breaks with precious metals not only acknowledges them, but also pays tribute to the vessel that has been torn apart by the mutability of life. The previously broken object is considered more beautiful for its imperfections. In life, too, even greater brilliance can be found after the mending.

As an emergency medicine physician, I know how to be still for others. I know how to call down the gods of repose and silence, to take the measure of their power in the moments when I need it most. This stillness I inhabit as I pause, push, breathe, and grow.

The stories I tell here will, I hope, take you into the chaos of emergency medicine and show you where the center is. This center is where we find the sturdy roots of insight that can't be windthrown by passing storms. In their grounding they offer nourishment that can, should we allow it, lead to lives of ever-increasing growth. I had to find this center for myself as I took stock of experiences that were exceedingly painful yet that ultimately filled me with the promise of a meaningful rebirth, a rebirth that is worth the surviving, worth the healing, worth the repair.

THE BEAUTY IN BREAKING

ONE

Michele: A Wing and a Prayer

I AM SEVEN AND A HALF. I am bathed in a quiet punctuated only by the rhythmic upsweeping whistle of the northern cardinal's song. It's almost never like this, but right now the only sound emerging from our three-bedroom Colonial is the refrigerator's hum. No one is screaming or yelling, no one is punching, no one is being hit, no piece of furniture has toppled to the floor. Today there are no new bruises and no new scars. It is Saturday afternoon and it is absolutely tranquil: My brother, sister, and father are out. My mother is down the hall in her room.

I gather up three of my favorite My Little Pony figurines, holding one in each hand and tucking one under my left arm, leave my bedroom, and walk downstairs. All I can hear is the whisper my socks make with each step on the hardwood floor.

After moving to Washington, DC, when I was four years old, my family proceeded to change homes three times within a four-mile distance; homes two and three were less than a mile apart. Each move was precipitated by my parents' desire to live in increasingly attractive homes in increasingly exclusive neighborhoods. It was a game whose prize was not comfort but prestige, so they bought and sold homes until they ultimately lost. This is home number two, on Sixteenth Street in Northwest Washington, close to the border with Silver Spring, Maryland.

I walk down the staircase that ends in the foyer, then through the foyer to the living room, and finally to the Fish Room, so named by my little sister and me for the large aquarium that is its centerpiece.

The people on my mother's side of the family were very superstitious. You don't walk under ladders. At all costs you avoid breaking a mirror. You always look at the new moon over your right shoulder. And you never *ever* split a pole. The fish tank fit neatly into this paradigm. As my parents explained, it was meant to activate positive chi and block the negative energy in an environment. The tank was home to a small array of tropical fish. Siamese fighting fish, whose fins were a rainbow of fiery plums giving way to reds, were always included in the aquarium selection. What seemed like every several weeks the fish would die, and then my parents would buy new ones, which would suffer the same fate. It struck me as strange that they simply replaced the fish without first conducting a thorough analysis on what had caused the aquatic massacre.

Today, as I enter the Fish Room, I note that the aquarium

(a thirty-gallon rectangular glass prism atop a simple, tall, black metal stand) has recently been replenished. Sun pours through the windowpanes, casting shadows on the butterscotch wood. I settle cross-legged on the floor and masterfully jockey my team of horses over each groove and shifting beam of light. They are skilled and graceful jumpers, but what else could be expected of ponies from a peaceful paradise estate?

Completely absorbed in the play, I feel an ease suffuse my entire being. For those cherished minutes, the armor that encases my spirit loosens and I am wholly open to the moment. Then, as if on Pegasus's wings, I feel a presence floating with me in the room, next to the red velvet sofa, in front of the fish tank, which faces the bay window. When I look for it, it is just me, alone in the softly lit room. I see no one, though I feel and hear a gentle essence. Her voice is so familiar that when she speaks, it's as if the words were my own.

Michele, you are okay. You will be okay. You will be safe. Your mother will be safe. Your brother and sister will be safe.

Security was perhaps the only thing I ever wanted, and up to that point it had remained a long-ungranted wish.

The benediction continues: *You will live. You must. Your mother will live. Your brother and sister will live. You will grow to see that you will help many people. You will grow to do great service. You must.*

I sit on the floor, the ponies strewn about me, momentarily forgotten. I feel my eyes widen more with each word. It is the stupor in the face of answered prayer, the astonishment of gratitude. For once, nothing in me is afraid. And just like that, as soon as she has arrived, she is gone. Just one message, and then she vanished.

I knew about guardian angels from TV shows. They are always visions in white gowns with expansive wings who float on beds of cumulus clouds. There was no visual for mine, just a voice that sounded clear and sure, an articulation that permeated the room. I can't contain my excitement—I fully believe this message has been from an angel. For the first time in my life I am spilling over with joy. I sprint upstairs to my mother to let her know that we will survive.

It is this very message that buttressed me for the next two decades of my life. On so many days, when all signs pointed away from my not only thriving but surviving, I remembered the angel's whispers and felt saved.

I cannot count how many times I longed to be rescued in my father's homes. The beauty of this one, on its large, tree-lined, and well-manicured lot, belied the chaos raging within.

You couldn't hear it from the street. Just the day before the angel came, I had been in my room with my sister, in the midst of a stuffed animal caucus, while our brother, John, was in his room, stereo blaring the latest '80s R&B hits. Then I felt my brother's door bang open and the floor shake as he sprinted down the stairs. My sister and I stopped cold and locked eyes. My blood curdled for a terrifying moment. I heard something wooden fall, feet scuffling across the floor downstairs, and a body thrown against a wall. Then my mother's scream—"Stop!"—was immediately cut off as she was strangled mute.

I had to go downstairs. I had to stop it. I had to help my older brother, who was on his way into the fray. I had to stop my father from killing my mother.

Honestly, I don't know what's worse: constructing an image of the brutality in your mind's eye or actually bearing witness to it. At seven, I didn't have the power to choose. At seven, you attach in the only way you know how: You think you love even the attacker, the one who hurts you and your family. At seven, you blame yourself. In that split second, as I waited, frozen in terror, I knew only that at any given time, everything I wanted and everything I cherished could be taken from me. I knew that I didn't deserve to be happy because although I couldn't understand what and I couldn't understand how or why, I knew that I must have done something terribly wrong. I knew that I had to run downstairs to save a life, but I couldn't face yet again the terror in which, somehow, I had played a pivotal role.

Seconds later, I was on the stairs, my younger sister right behind me. Toward the bottom, she stopped short and lost her balance, causing her to accidentally nudge me farther down. I clung to the banister to keep from falling. We stood there, afraid to enter the scene.

After summoning my courage, I walked into the kitchen to see my mother standing alone, bracing herself against the wall. My brother stood in the middle of the room. Two chairs and a broom were strewn across the floor, and shards of shattered glass were everywhere. My father was gone, and the front door was wide-open.

"Be careful, girls. Don't step on the glass! Go get shoes!" my mother cried out, gasping.

My brother walked over to the chairs and began to right them.

"Oh my, I've lost my earring. Dern!" my mother exclaimed. It was an allowable expletive employed by my grandparents. My mother's parents were Southern, so this was likely the regional variation of "darn."

"Where in the world is that earring?" my mother continued, acting as if that were the most important detail of the scene we confronted. For her, it was.

My sister had already gone upstairs, put on shoes, and was now hard at work peering into every nook and cranny of the kitchen.

My mother picked up the broom and began sweeping up the glass. "Careful, kids, watch where you step. Gosh, I hope I don't sweep up that earring."

I, too, retrieved my shoes and returned to help. I went to the open front door and looked outside. There was no one. In keeping with my indoctrination, I closed the door firmly to seal the secrets inside.

Within minutes, my sister had found the sapphire stud earring that had rolled under the corner of the Oriental rug in the foyer.

"My goodness, how did it get over there?" my mother asked. "I knew it—good old Eagle Eyes gets it again! Thank you, my darling." She plucked the earring from my sister's small palm and gave her a hug. "I'll find another backing. That's less important. I must have an extra upstairs."

She put the earring on the counter so she could finish sweeping up the glass. As she bent toward the dustpan, her hair fell forward, and when she brushed it back, I could see red marks on her neck. The nail of her index finger was broken, and the ragged edge was covered in dried blood. She winced a little as the pressure from the dustpan dug into her bruised finger.

My brother balled up his fists and silently climbed the stairs—a moment later I heard him resume listening to his latest vinyl album: Prince's *Purple Rain*. While my sister sat quivering with my mother in the kitchen, I went into the foyer and sat on the bottom step of the staircase. I waited in the event my father returned. I waited in case my sister cried. I waited for my fluttering heart to be still. I waited even after my mother had put the broom away, retrieved her sapphire earring from the counter, and walked past me to go upstairs to her room. I waited for the discussion our family would never have.

And, really, what kind of discussion would it have been? Would we have all gathered in the living room, we three children on the sofa and a parent seated at either end in antique chairs?

If he were to have spoken the truth, here is what my father would have said:

I come from a place of deep shame and self-loathing. I never learned to forgive my parents for abandoning me, so I never learned to love. Instead of taking the time to heal from my past traumas, I chose to distract myself by marrying before I was fit to be in a relationship of any kind. Every day, by not making a better choice, the right choice, I choose to tether myself to this dysfunction. Because of this, I have made a choice to continue that cycle of pain and suffering. For this reason, I have decided to rob myself of health and genuine connection. For this same reason, I choose to terrorize you and rob you of any sense of security and childhood. It won't stop until decades from now, when I finally walk out of your lives. And yes, I know that I am wrong. It's true that I should have committed none of this violence. You will or will not find your own closure as you wish. You will or will not find your own healing as you wish. As for me, I will run from this place. I will hide from myself beneath the cloak of Christianity. I will let these silent compartments of denial and hurt imprison me in this life. That hell is my temple.

In turn, my mother would have said the following:

I learned in my formative years to be codependent and so never truly developed the tenor of my own voice. I tell myself I am helping a broken man. What I'm really doing is finding someone to validate my low self-esteem, then imprinting that dysfunction onto the next generation. I fill up this void with fancy, attractive possessions. I found a man who can give us things. Don't you all want nice things? I realize that when you children finally escape this house, you will not know what it means to sleep through the night without fear. You will not know what it means to love from a place of absolute self-possession. It will be up to you later to decide if and how you will learn these skills on your own. As for me, I will allow all this to lay the groundwork for me to live a smaller life than I ever wanted for myself or for my children. I can't face my own pain. I can't face that my inaction to make a better choice, the right choice, has led to the harm of myself and my children. It is true that I should have left . . . And yet, I choose to stay here now in spite of it all. Be well, my children, be well.

Here is what I would have said to both of them:

Speak these truths aloud, for it is only in silence that horror can persist. The courage to call a thing by its true name galvanizes the human spirit to address it. If that condition serves one's desires, it will be embraced with a full heart. If it is destructive to one's path, it will be deliberately dismantled over time.

And so it was that instead of facing the truth of our demons, my family went on in silence year after year, our days routinely punctuated by bursts of violence. After an argument over something mundane—who had misplaced the car keys, who would pick up the girls after school—my father threw punches at my mother. Over time, my brother, John, whom my classmates regarded as if he were a part-time print model and part-time professional athlete, grew into a muscular man of five foot ten with the physical power to intervene. My father was just shorter than the average American male, and fat: It was his emotional instability and not his build that was intimidating. John would pull my father off my mother and then the two men would begin to tussle.

Once, in my early teenage years, I flung myself into an argument that my father and my brother were having in an effort to protect John, but as I was just five feet tall and weighed not even one hundred pounds, I grossly misgauged my strength. When a punch careened against my arm, I was thrown back onto the floor. My mother screamed for me to move out of the way and for my father to stop. John then flipped atop my father to wrestle him into submission, every muscle in his young body pinning the madman to the floor. I scooted back and ran to my room for some type of weapon. Could I use a book or one of my larger troll dolls to pummel my father? What if I missed him and hit my brother? What if that gave the monster the advantage and then none of us would be safe? Yes, I thought about calling the police, but in that neighborhood, you didn't call the police on your own family.

With the final DC home, house number three, we had arrived on the "Gold Coast." Areas colloquially referred to as the Gold and Platinum Coasts of Washington, DC, were so named because they were historically home to Washington's black elite. I landed there in the fourth grade with a new status, at a new private school for girls, the National Cathedral School. Like all elites, we didn't expose our private, upper-middle-class shame to the public sphere. Why would we have? After all, we had worked too hard to get here to risk a crack in the fragile façade that fronted our legitimacy. All elites knew the code: Take your pills with your cocktail, use your cosmetics to cover the blemishes and bruises, clean up quickly, whatever it takes so you can present a smiling, perfectly coiffed and clad self to the world.

I broke this code of privilege only once. I was a tween when, one Saturday afternoon, I fled the melee in the second-floor master bedroom where my teenage brother was fighting my father to protect my mother and as my mother was fighting my father on the periphery to defend my brother, and my sister was somewhere unidentifiable but not visibly in the fray. I ran downstairs to the phone docked on the wall outside the kitchen. Tucked in the dark where no one would see me, I desperately dialed.

I heard: "Nine-one-one. What is your emergency?"

"I'm at home. We're not safe. My father is hitting my mother. He's fighting with my brother. We're not safe here!" I whispered into the phone.

"Where are you located?" the voice asked.

I looked around and, with my hand over my mouth, stealthily told them where I was calling from and what was happening.

"We'll send a unit right out to you," the operator said.

"Please, please hurry," I begged before hanging up.

I ran upstairs to my parents' room. As my father and brother fought and my mother swatted my father with her shoe, I managed to yell out, "I've called the police. They're on their way!"

This was my leverage. The beating stopped, but the

threats continued to fly. My father threatened to have my brother arrested. My mother retorted that she would never allow such a thing and that it was my father who should be arrested.

They were still arguing when the doorbell rang. I ran downstairs to open the front door. Two male DC police officers were standing there. They adjusted their gaze down from the iron grate peephole to see a little girl framed in the doorway. One officer had a hand on his holster; the other officer stood with his arms crossed. As if in stereo, they fired off rounds of questions at me.

"Did anyone here call nine-one-one?"

"What seems to be the problem?"

"Is there a disturbance here?"

"We received a call about a domestic dispute."

I opened my mouth to reply, but standing on the doorstep looking out into my quiet, placid neighborhood, I found the answers hard, so hard, to utter. I saw the police car parked on the street in front of my house. I wondered if the Fraziers, next door, were home. I wondered if Sammy, my crush who lived around the corner, would ride by on his bike and see the police car and me with my side ponytail and favorite striped dress. At least I was well dressed, I thought, for my unexpected guests and any unsuspecting onlookers.

"Miss," the police officer on the left said, jolting me back to attention. "Did you call the police?"

It was as if he had asked me to recite the complete value of pi. I could have given him a basic idea of its beginning, but

I had no idea in what order it unfolded and no clue about how it might end. I could feel my breathing accelerate as I thought about what I might say, but then the adults rushed to the door, whisking me aside.

I stood in the corner of the foyer as my mother, brother, and father spoke to the police. As far as I could hear, each of them was frantically interjecting his or her version of the story. Emboldened by the police presence, my sister and I chimed in to corroborate our team's account.

The police listened quietly and with little patience. Finally, they said, "Well, if you all want to stay with your stories, we'll just have to arrest you both," indicating both my father and brother.

I could feel my sister's heart sink with my own. How had these officers parsed the blame to dismantle justice in this way? How did my father's account equal the collective account of us four? How had my call yielded their indifference instead of assistance, which was yet another punishing blow?

My mother spoke up right away, her voice filled with dread. "No, no, no, I don't want my son arrested"—and because she couldn't risk my brother being jailed, she then said she didn't want to press any charges against my father, either.

And that was the end of the police involvement. The two officers looked at my parents and, without saying anything else, turned and went back to their cruiser.

After they left, I realized that there really wasn't anyone we could turn to. There was no law here. No help. When assessing the danger, the police had not differentiated between my father and my brother. They had not asked me or my sister if we were safe. Without so much as a verbal censure to my father, they had simply abandoned a woman and her children to a clear danger in their house.

Worse perhaps, I had broken the code of how "good" families behave, only to find that traditional avenues would neither protect nor serve me.

We never spoke of the 911 call—no one ever mentioned it—and I never dialed those three numbers again. When my parents fought—and they continued to—I just prayed to my angel that it would all end well one day. And one gorgeous fall day years later, it did end—in a way. Or maybe it is more accurate to say that on that gorgeous fall day to come, I was able to see a way out.

Years after I called the police, the usual battle was raging as I cowered in my room, contemplating, once again, what I might use as a weapon to protect myself and my family against my father. Then I heard someone leave the house, the door slamming shut. My father had stormed upstairs and thrown clothes in a bag. He then got his car keys and left the house without saying a word, driving away for what all of us hoped would be forever but collectively knew would be for only a few days.

I hesitantly emerged into the hallway. My mother stood there holding my brother's hand; he was bleeding from a deep wound in his left thumb. Our father had bitten him while John had had him pinned to the floor.

As my mother ripped the hem of John's frayed shirt to

fashion a makeshift tourniquet to stop the bleeding, I couldn't help but wonder: What kind of animal bites a fellow human being, his own son, like this?

Amid the chaos, we pressed on with the other versions of our lives. My mother needed to drive my sister to a friend's birthday party. Since I had recently obtained my learner's permit, I volunteered to take my brother to the closest ER we could think of, a ten-minute drive away, in Silver Spring. My mother agreed, and the four of us dispersed in two cars.

As I drove my burnished tan Corolla, it was hard to avoid staring at the bandaged hand resting in my brother's lap. When we arrived at the hospital, I followed the red arrows to the circular driveway for the emergency department drop-off area. My brother had to reach across his lap with his un-injured hand to liberate himself from the seat belt before getting out of the car.

I watched him start the long walk toward the fluorescent lights beckoning from the ER and then I drove around to the hospital parking lot. I parked and got out of the car, hud-dling into my sweater as I took note of the majestic maple and elm trees beside the stoic pines that remained forever green along the path toward the imposing gray high-rise. I belted my sweater and headed inside. In stark contrast to the chill of the bright white ER lights, the hospital entrance was warm and dark.

It was quiet inside, and I saw no one walking the shiny linoleum floors. I found my brother in the waiting room fill-ing out some forms, and I took a seat next to him. An older man sat at the other end of the room, his hair disheveled and his skin creased from what even at my young age looked like a lifetime of hard living. He had pulled his heavy brown trench coat over him as he slept in the unyielding waiting room chair, his head bobbing with each big-bellied breath. For long moments at a time he would stop breathing altogether, and I found myself watching anxiously until he took another breath. I figured that if the next one didn't come, at least he was in an ER.

A young man was sitting in a chair toward the middle of the room with his discharge papers, an inhaler, and a bottle of medicine. He kept looking out toward the parking lot, and I gathered he was waiting for a ride. The ER doors slid open, and a father hurried in carrying his little girl, who had a nasty gash on her leg just below the hem of her purple dress.

All of us were there, I realized, because we were damaged in some way. Wounded. Broken.

A few minutes later, my brother was called into the inner recesses of the ER. I watched him disappear into a triage area and then out of view. I settled in for the wait.

Flashing lights and high-pitched beeps pierced the lull, announcing the arrival of an ambulance backing up to the ER doors. The vehicle parked, and then the crew proceeded to unload a portly older man lying on a gurney. A medic held up a bag of fluid that dripped into the man's arm. He secured it to a metal pole and then continued to pump air into a tube that went into the man's mouth. Another medic performed compressions on the man's chest, but the man did not move, save for the intermittent involuntary jerking of his body in time with the thrusts to his chest. At one point, an ashen arm dangled off the gurney as they rushed the patient into the emergency department.

Moments later, what appeared to be a family flooded into the waiting room: Women and men came in crying, asking about their father, husband, son. The clerk at the intake desk quietly asked them to wait. I picked up a magazine and tried not to stare as wounded people came in, nurses arrived to call out names, patients walked or were wheeled into rooms, and curtains closed around their beds. The wounded little girl, the old man, the family—the whole gamut of life seemed to be converging in this space.

All of us sat there waiting, nervously averting our eyes from one another. At one point, a burgundy car pulled up outside and the young man with the inhaler and discharge papers exclaimed, "Finally! Thank God!" gathered his belongings, and rushed for the door. The old man under the overcoat, who I decided must be homeless, continued to sleep. The family members, still crying, eventually were ushered into an interior room. The little girl with the gash on her leg skipped out, hand in hand with her father, wearing a brand-new pink Band-Aid and clutching a lollipop; she was smiling as if she'd just been to the circus.

I glanced at my watch: It had been slightly over an hour and there was still no sign of my brother. Later, the family of the man who'd arrived by ambulance came out one by one, arm in arm, shaking their heads and wringing their hands. As they headed out into the night, there was talk of arrangements and who would call Aunt Jo.

Now it was just me and the Sleeper. Dusk set in as I continued to wait. Finally, my brother emerged, his hand bandaged in thick white gauze. He was ready to go.

"How is everything?" I asked

"Fine. They just did an X-ray and cleaned it up. I have to have it checked in a couple of days to make sure it's healing all right. They said something about how they could only put a couple of stitches since it's a bad bite wound, and I have to take these antibiotics."

As my brother and I left the ER, I marveled at the place, one of bright lights and dark hallways, a place so quiet and yet so throbbing with life. I marveled at how a little girl could be carried in cut and crying and then skip out laughing; at how a bloodied brother could reappear with stitches in his repaired hand; at how the family of a man who had presumably been fine that morning could manage to leave without him to start a new stage of their lives, one in which he would play no part; at how the man without a home could find somewhere to rest until he, too, would have to go back outside to figure out the rest of his day, the rest of his life; at how all of us had converged in these hallowed halls for a chance to reveal our wounds, to offer up our hurt and our pain to be eased. If my brother's body could be patched up, then certainly, in its own time, his spirit could mend, too. If we looked, if we named the problem, identified and examined it, then there was the opportunity to fix it, the chance for us to walk out under the stoic pines healed, or on our way to being so.

On the drive home, my brother and I assumed our usual silence. The city at dusk was cloaked in shadows, and the full moon played mischief among the clouds. I pulled my Toyota into our driveway behind my mother's Lincoln Town Car and alongside my brother's sports car. We went into the house, and John headed up to his room and turned on his music—this time A Tribe Called Quest. I went into the kitchen and poured myself a glass of orange juice, then sat at the kitchen table and thought about how I wanted to leave this haunted house and fix people. I figured that if I could find stillness in this chaos, if I could find love beyond this violence, if I could heal these layers of wounds, then I would be the doctor in my own emergency room. That would be my offering to the world, to myself. Unlike in the war zone that was my childhood, I would be in control of that space, providing relief or at least a reprieve to those who called out for help. I would see to it that there was shelter in the spaces of which I was the guardian. The formless angel with a voice as clear as my own had told me the secret many years ago. Let it be so.

TWO

Dr. Harper:
The View from Here

IT WASN'T AT ALL how I had pictured graduation from my emergency medicine residency at Mercy Hospital in the South Bronx would be, but it certainly was a blistering end. I sat near the aisle, next to my mother, who was next to my stepfather. I had told my brother and sister not to bother with the trip. I figured my sister would be busy with her obligations as an army lieutenant. I assumed that my brother would be preoccupied with his family or with landscaping his new home. That's what I told myself. The truth was closer to my not wanting them to see me like this. I didn't want witnesses there to confirm that this had really happened, that this celebration I had looked forward to for the last four years of medical school, and then during the four years of residency, felt more like a funeral. There was a noticeable absence by my side, where I had always imagined my husband would have stood.

Husband. The word cut like a slur.

Ex-husband was more accurate. The last time I spent time with Dan was in May, in our twelve-hundred-square-foot, two-bedroom prewar co-op in the South Bronx. Our marriage was unmistakably over, but we had continued co-habitating because my move to Pennsylvania was still more than one month away, just after graduation. (Neither Dan nor I had the money for another place at that time with the sale of our co-op still pending.)

We had previously settled on Philadelphia. Our families were in the Northeast, and we were Northeasterners at heart. New York City was too expensive, anything north of New York was too cold, and anything south of DC was no longer the North. Most of New Jersey was far too suburban, and the parts that offered big-city comforts were just as expensive as New York City. This had left only Philadelphia, which had easy access to New York, DC, New Jersey, and Maryland, and had a reasonable cost of living compared to its competition. Neither one of us had ever lived there, but it seemed to make the most sense on paper. I didn't know anyone in Philadelphia, but Dan's parents had just moved to one of its bedroom communities, and he had a couple of friends who lived nearby.

We had deferred every other decision until after my residency—when one member of a couple is in residency, the couple is in residency—but now all that would change. In our new city, I had imagined we would walk over cobblestone streets hand in hand. Ginkgo leaves would waft gently onto the sidewalks as we passed. We'd try all the new restaurants because we'd finally be able to afford them. I couldn't wait to advertise all our starter IKEA furniture on *Craigslist* and purchase the type of furniture an adult woman actually *wanted* to pack up and take with her when she relocated. Our home's style would be a mix of elegant and eco-industrial. We'd burn candles all the time, vanilla and spiced amber to start. We'd finally have placemats, napkins, and sleek new flatware. We'd wander the city museums on Wednesdays and host dinner parties on Fridays. We'd enjoy our discretionary income and then, after a couple of years, we could discuss having kids.

So our split could have been a scene from a terrible indie film, the one where the perfect, young, progressive New York City couple—the white independent filmmaker husband and the black physician wife who had met at Harvard's freshman ice-cream social—endure a shocking, painful breakup. The couple has already overcome so much when, only months before she graduates from her residency, with a planned move to Philadelphia to be near his friends and family, he lowers the boom.

"You're doing well in your career, and I'm not," he told me that night. "If I'm with you, I'll focus on your success. I have to find myself. The only way I can do that is if I'm not with you. You'll be fine in Philadelphia. I can't go."

It felt like a cliché, a plot point that everybody else but the main characters themselves sees coming.

I knew what would happen next in the movie. It would

start raining outside—first a drizzle and then a torrential downpour, as Whitney Houston crooned "I Will Always Love You." As the music grew louder, I would rest my head on his shoulder. Then, as the song reached its crescendo, my heart would break.

In real life, forty-eight hours after his declaration, I found an attorney and filed for divorce.

We had talked until three o'clock in the morning, our words alternating between clench-fisted blame and gut-wrenching pleas. We had paced miles in that bedroom, until our bodies broke from fatigue. Finally, we had collapsed into bed. I tossed and turned the rest of the night away, unable to dispel the slideshow of snapshots that was our story—well, *my* version of our story. I knew that time would fade each image to a hazy déjà vu.

I begged the universe to make me remember our cheesy romantic dancing in the rain on a temperate April afternoon nine years before; our special Queens hummus recipe we had concocted from a handful of Food Network recipes and whatever happened to be our flavor preference of the week; our road trips to the Jersey Shore; his touch, which was smooth and soft in the way of a person whose work is more cognitive than physical; the brown pools of his eyes that told me that beneath his athletic build, he was fragile; and every second of the thirteen years we had shared. I begged the universe to make our breakup feel fair or right, and to let me survive.

I had attempted to soothe myself by crawling up close

and snuggling into him. I lay there in the nook made by his arms, timing my breath to the heavy breath of his sleep, the rhythmic calm of his presence. (Dan had always had this gift: He could sleep anytime, anywhere.) His sculpted body felt supple as the muscle softened in slumber, providing the perfect cushion for bite-size me. I'm still amazed at how the body yields when it relaxes. I don't know if it was because, in true *Iron Chef* fashion, he frequently whipped up fresh Italian dishes with whatever ingredients were on hand, or because of his long days running around the New York City streets for his film shoots, but that night, Dan smelled like a mixture of warm bread and grass. I inhaled deeply, as if it were the most precious breath I would ever take. I felt as if I were levitating there, as if in a hot-air balloon going up, up, up. I wanted so badly to come down, to snuggle closer, but there was a rampart of air, of breath, between us.

I looked over the edge of the balloon's wicker basket and waved good-bye to this place. I thought of our earlier plan, before we knew we were breaking up, to rent out the co-op as an investment property when we moved to Philadelphia, until the real estate market swelled to secure us a hefty sale price. It was our surefire way to get rich, we had mused.

As the balloon kept rising, I panned the landscape to catch a glimpse of my in-laws and silently bade them good-bye, too. It had taken them nearly a decade to become comfortable with their baby boy dating a black woman, with their having a black daughter-in-law. In the end, it was worth it: Our bond had weathered strong. The thought of my relocating to their area without their son made the pang of my move that much more acute.

I said my farewells, too, to the two beautiful, olive-skinned, kinky-haired children Dan and I might have had. I could still feel the curls that framed their cherubic cheeks, which had my dimples. Their Italian American and African American heritages would have blessed them with lean, muscular bodies and round, ample butts. She would have been Nella Vita, and he would have been August. I could hear their giggles and their bye-byes dissolving into shrieks and cries. I tried to hold on to their images, but the balloon was drifting too high, and I was receding from them and my in-laws and the apartment and everything else I had known for the past thirteen years.

Now the balloon was up too far for me to jump down. The air felt thin at this altitude, and the only bubble of oxygen was right there on my ex-husband's chest and neck. My eyes traced his every contour—the mandible, the clavicle, the iliac crest—because I knew it would be the last time. I knew that at some point, he would wake up, and I would have to move. Trembling, I fumbled for my phone to snap one last picture of him asleep in bed. It was a terrible photo: The image was blurry and, in the low light, sepia-toned. I couldn't help but laugh, anticipating his response when I showed it to him after he woke—unless, of course, I simply deleted it.

Soon, a sticky New York City spring morning dawned.

Sunrise oozed through the blinds and sketched a pattern on Dan's left cheek. I peeled the sheet back to feel the shallow breeze of the fan as it fought a pathetic battle against the humidity, and I thought about my next step.

I would fall apart.

Part of it would be due to loneliness, and a greater part would be the loss of what had been, up to that point, the only relatively stable relationship I had ever had with a man.

I wasn't angry the marriage was over. I wasn't bitter. I knew that we had run our course. Our breakup had never really been about the moving; it had been about two people at a crossroads. Dan wanted to live abroad to study his craft, knowing full well that I couldn't move after my residency. I needed to start working and to pass my board certification examination. He knew that I was not the type of woman to kamikaze my career for a man. I was also not the type of woman to stand in the way of another person's path. For Dan's part, he would leave because he had to. And I would let him go because there was no question that I had to.

No, the sadness on its way was over something greater than loneliness or "losing a man." The breakup of my marriage was stoking in me the deep sense of abandonment that had lain dormant during my marriage, the loss of the home life I had craved but never had. I knew on some level that *this* was the real source of my grief.

I didn't know the details yet—how or when—but that New York City spring, I knew it wouldn't be long before I

slipped into a well of despondence, one where there was neither color nor light, but where, goddess willing, there was a
bottom. I knew, too, that there would be no fighting any of it.

Now, here at my final residency ceremony, I shifted in my
seat and glanced at my mother as she proudly anticipated my
name being called. I concentrated on the rhythmic tapping
of my heel. Just a few minutes more in this auditorium and I
could start the business of moving on. I was careful not to
kick the stranger beside me, to make the tapping fine and
swift so it wouldn't bother anyone but could still distract
me. I looked down at my ring finger—I could still see the
light tan mark where my wedding band had been, the skin
around it darkened by the sun. I quickly rubbed my index
finger over the area. I rubbed it to take away the pain, and I
kept rubbing, hard, as a single errant tear seared my right
cheek. The strategy wasn't working.

Every graduation had sucked in its own way. High school
graduation had sucked the least. The ceremony itself was
revelrous. My whole family attended—no great feat, given
that my family is small. Grandma showed up in one of her
lacy church hats, which was nicely complemented by her
deep berry lipstick. Grandpa, taciturn and smiling, was
there in a smart suit, his camera, as always, by his side. He
was the family photographer and the consummate observer.
Grandma was the matriarch and the voice for them both. My
mother's favorite sister, Eileen, was there, and my parents,

my brother, and my sister, cheering with the rest of those gathered at the commencement for the National Cathedral School. The feeling of being surrounded by my fellow class-mates, sixty-six other young women, many of whom would undoubtedly alter the course of history in critical ways, gave me unparalleled pride.

So, high school graduation itself wasn't bad. Leaving my family home for college was the bittersweet bit: The place was all I had known as a little girl, and yet nearly everything about it had been wrong. As I packed, listening to Deee-lite on my CD player, I took with me my inner child. The girl I was, who had never been permitted to come out to explore and be fanciful and weightless. Tucked into a small box, I carried her on the long drive to Cambridge, Massachusetts, because outside of the Orchid Street walls she might finally find a playground.

I won't go into detail about my college experience. Much has been written about centers of elitism and privilege like Harvard University. Some of it is true. It is true that at one of the first social events at Harvard I attended, a white male classmate told me that I couldn't possibly be black because I didn't speak like the two black people he knew from his neighborhood—and since he was, clearly, the arbiter of "blackness" he felt he had the right to say that to me. What I didn't know at the time was that this would be a fitting intro-duction to the four years of micro- (well, really, macro-) ag-gressions to follow. It is true that when a student sexual violence prevention group I was a part of approached one of the deans with a multipoint plan, her response to our inquiry to centralize resources for rape victims was "Harvard doesn't hold your hand." She meant it. In less than the time it took for her to close her door, the discussion was over. It is true that when I heard of the scandal of wealthy people literally purchasing their children's admissions into these universities, I wasn't surprised—this rampant inequity was well-known to all of us who were there; the only thing bizarre about the story was that the public behaved as if they weren't aware. While these ivory towers have traditionally served to elevate those who already have unearned privilege, they may hinder those who do not, by virtue of immutable attributes such as color, family class, sexual orientation, gender, and physical ability. The increased scrutiny on these institutions to live up to the standards of conduct that they profess to exemplify is warranted.

As for the graduation ceremony itself, suffice it to say that various people gave speeches and I skipped the majority of the events.

It was my graduation from medical school that was a complete derealization. It wasn't just that my grandparents were no longer able to travel—my grandmother had developed advanced Alzheimer's, and my grandfather had stayed at home to care for the woman who had always anchored his world—but that Morris, my biological father, attended. He had been at all the graduations that came before, and it had been awkward each and every time. Up to that point, he had helped pay for my education, so I had felt obligated to extend the invitation. (I didn't yet know that I had the power to choose.) By the time I entered medical school, my parents had been divorced several years, which had made my conversations with my father sporadic and forced. I watched Morris shake hands with my instructors and tuned out his recounting of the nurturing fathering that he didn't do. As we posed for family photos, a tension in me snapped: Each camera flash documented that the charade my family had always been was now publicly foisted onto this next stage of my life, where it was neither welcome nor tolerable.

Soon after I finished medical school, Dan and I got married. I had promised my mother I wouldn't get married until after I'd earned my medical degree. As she had told me many times, she wanted me to own my degree all by myself. I had decided not to invite Morris to the marriage celebration; in fact, he didn't even know about it. Not long after, he let me know that he no longer wanted to be a part of my life. This was during one of the many phone conversations he coerced from me, asserting some type of genetic imperative to maintain a connection to one's family. When that failed, he'd try to control me with threats to withdraw financial support. When that failed—I decided that accepting his money came at far too high a cost—the coercion stopped. As far as I was concerned, the title of "father" had to be earned, and I began to define "family" for myself, concluding that inclusion in this group could be forfeited.

I cut these cords to support myself. I knew by then that it was only from that space that I could make my own assessments. It was only then that I could finally confront him about his abusive behavior. I told him that he had been a terrorist in our family, that he had so profoundly ruined some of its members' lives that they struggled with substance abuse, that my mother still flinched at loud noises. I told him that if he ever wanted to communicate with me again, he would first have to acknowledge the truth of who he was.

Instead of admitting that any of what I'd said had even occurred, he vanished. He made his choice.

It is better to be left with a ghost than a ghoul, so his disappearance from my life was an acceptable outcome.

There was no graduation from my internship, just an escape. My four-year emergency medicine program required that I complete my intern year (postgraduate year one of residency) in another field before returning to complete years two through four in the ER. The thinking in the profession at the time was that it was too tough to start off in the ER fresh out of medical school, that it was better to get a year of training under your belt in another medical discipline first. Figuring it would give me a well-rounded foundation for my practice in emergency medicine, I elected to spend my intern year in internal medicine. I almost didn't care where I completed that first year—for me, it was simply a 365-day means to an end. Still, I decided to diminish the pain by choosing a program with the relatively higher pay and other creature comforts a wealthy hospital affords. I therefore dutifully completed that year in a prosperous area of Long Island, at a hospital where, upon entering each day, I was greeted with a classical selection from the pianist seated at the grand piano in the lobby or from a serenading harpist.

(I had not anticipated that even this would not quell my longing every single day for my next medical home, in the Bronx.)

Internship is the year of residency that nearly everyone in medicine programs hates. Whether it was other prelims like me, who counted down the minutes until we arrived at our primary program; or the sad souls who hadn't yet been matched with a residency program but who had accepted the position in the hope that it would buy them some time as they scrambled to reapply to a residency; or the folks who actually wanted to practice internal medicine and so swallowed the bitter pill of the first year and accepted its drudgery as conventional hazing—we were, after all, the scut slaves of the hospital. The first to be paged for everything, we ran around chasing electrolyte levels, refilling Tylenol orders, and preparing morning presentations—just a fraction of the duties we performed on minimal sleep.

The internal medicine program director I worked under, Dr. Jaiswal, was a forceful character. She was intelligent and skilled clinically, but not particularly nice. As we interns gathered for rounds, the morning ritual where we visited patients to check on their progress, we always knew when she was approaching by the *click-clack* of her shoes on the linoleum. She matched her sensible yet stylish kitten heels with jewel-toned suits that always seemed to be at least one size too large for her petite frame.

One summer morning, after I had been on call the night before, we would be starting with my presentation of patient signs and symptoms followed by the prescribed evaluation and treatment plans for anyone I had admitted overnight—at which point, I could go home to rest while the others on the team continued with rounds. The day before, Dr. Jaiswal had reamed out Helen, another one of the prelims, for her presentation on pneumonia, and Craig for his feeble attempt to present a patient with thrombocytopenia (low platelet count) in view of everyone in the vicinity of the doctors' stations where we were rounding. Everyone feared Dr. Jaiswal, harboring a resentment toward her that bordered on hate. In the resident lounge, the comments made about her were brutal, and we complained incessantly to one another about how overly critical she was and how stingy with positive feedback.

While Dr. Jaiswal was less than forgiving of careless intern error, I had to admit that she was probably on point with her criticisms of Helen and Craig: Their presentations had been weak. And in her defense, she could tell you everything about her patients. For example, Dr. Jaiswal knew that Mr. Jones, who had been brought to the hospital in multiorgan failure, had suffered a botched knee replacement five years earlier. Fearing another bad hospital experience, he waited at home for three weeks with increasing knee pain and swelling before he allowed his family to call EMS to transport him to the ER for his septic joint. Also, she was a good diagnostician, and had even spotted in one patient acute intermittent porphyria, a disease rarely ever considered outside Discovery Health Channel's *Mystery Diagnosis* or the movie *The Madness of King George*. And though she was brusque, if you could absorb her example, you had every chance of becoming a phenomenal clinician. Tenderness would have to be learned elsewhere.

On that uncomfortable summer morning in my first month of intern year, it was my turn. As our medical team headed to my patient's room, I felt myself getting light-headed from a mix of sleep deprivation and fear. The walk from the fifth floor felt like a sprint. We were already on the seventh floor as if by time travel. Had we gotten on an elevator? I shuffled my papers, willing myself to remember everything I had learned about the patient the night before. (Dr. Jaiswal berated us if we glanced down at our notes during a presentation. Her logic: If we couldn't retain the information on a couple of patients at a time, then we had chosen the wrong field.) Nervously, I reminded myself of what I knew: The patient had a history of high cholesterol and hypertension. He was on no medications other than Crestor, for his cholesterol.

"So, Michele," Dr. Jaiswal said to me as we made our way to his room. "I hear you enjoyed a quiet evening. How lucky for you! Only one admission for us this morning? Well, we'll make the most of it!" She smiled, baring even, white teeth behind matte crimson lips. (She always wore red lipstick, and the hue seemed to amplify her every word.)

Quiet? Had she just used the word *quiet?* When I'd walked into the hospital last night, it was as if I were walking the plank. Just three other interns and I were covering the ward, and I felt the usual dread of holding other people's lives in my not-yet-capable hands. Two of my patients spiked fevers, one became hypoxic, one had chest pain, and another went into a rapid heart rate, which made me go into an even faster arrhythmia. There was nothing about the evening that had felt quiet, and now I didn't feel "lucky," either.

We reached the door to the patient's room and gathered around. I cleared my throat and began to present. "Mr. Frame is—"

"Oh, no, no, no," Dr. Jaiswal said. "Let's go in. Let us *see* the patient. Very important to actually go to the bedside and see the patient you are caring for. Assessment starts at first glance."

She couldn't be serious. Not only did I have to present to Dr. Jaiswal after I had been up all night, but I had to do so *in front of the patient?* As Dr. Jaiswal ushered the team inside the room, there was no time for me to anticipate the myriad ways this could all go terribly wrong. With a swiping motion of her finger, she indicated where each of us, obedient sheep that we were, should stand around the bed.

"Good morning, Mr. Frame," she said to the patient.

"I'm Dr. Jaiswal, the head of the medicine team who will be taking care of you. I hope you don't mind that we will be discussing your care right here with you."

"Not at all. Nice to meet you all," Mr. Frame responded. He was a nondescript, middle-aged white man with dark hair and a medium build. The spotlight of my having to discuss him to my supervising physician at his bedside gave him a new level of distinction.

"Hello, again," I said, nodding to the patient.

Then I began anew: "Mr. Frame is a fifty-nine-year-old male with a history of hypertension and high cholesterol with a chief complaint of worsening fevers, chills, cough, and nausea who was admitted with a liver abscess. He had been treated for this with two courses of antibiotics before coming to us. He completed a ten-day course of Augmentin, and then his primary care provider changed him to a course of Clindamycin. He was on day seven of ten when he presented last night."

"Dr. Harper, this already sounds very strange. Who was treating him?" Dr. Jaiswal asked.

"His primary care provider."

"Just his primary care provider? Huh. And what was he being treated for?"

"As I understand it, it was for a liver abscess, until his doctor sent him into the hospital last night." In my mind I scrolled through my notes, but I feared they wouldn't help. I didn't know. I hadn't adequately reasoned through the case. "Um, yes, I seem to remember that it was only his primary care provider who had been treating him before he came in last evening."

"Does that strike you as odd? Why would his primary care provider take this course of action to treat him, as a sole provider, with only oral antibiotics for a liver abscess? There's something missing here, something missing in the history. It simply doesn't make sense." Dr. Jaiswal paused as if to give me space for an impossible redemption.

I could hear each intern's bated breath and the rustle of Mr. Frame's crisp white hospital sheets as he shifted in bed. The air was humid and stale with the smell of half-eaten toast from the breakfast tray at the foot of his roommate's bed. In the hallway, nurses opened and closed cabinet drawers for the morning medication administration. The housekeeping staff knocked on doors asking permission to clear trash. Against the backdrop of this din, I stood in the cramped room in front of a ring of interns and our resident, floundering for answers I didn't have.

Finally, I spoke. "Well, the patient had a fever with his infection and continued to have fevers through the Augmentin, so the physician changed him to Clindamycin."

"Huh? What testing had been done prior to his presentation?" she asked.

"As I gathered from his history, lab, and radiology results the patient brought with him, his primary care doctor had completed blood work consisting of a CBC [complete blood count], basic metabolic panel, blood cultures, and also a chest X-ray. There was a persistent elevation in his white count and a small pleural effusion on the chest X-ray."

Dr. Jaiswal grimaced. "Uh-huh. Dr. Harper, you are *clearly* missing some critical information as well as basic medical knowledge, which has degraded your presentation and assessment here. Proceed for now, and we will get back to it," she directed.

I shook off my terror and continued. "Chest CT in the ER last night demonstrated a pleural effusion as well as a collection in the liver. A dedicated CT of his abdomen and pelvis was pursued to further evaluate this finding, which revealed his hepatic abscess."

"Yes, now it's making more sense," Dr. Jaiswal stated. "Sounds like there was no diagnosis apart from fever of unknown or at least unclear etiology and some nonspecific small pleural effusion found on a chest X-ray as the PCP worked up the patient. Due to Mr. Frame's worsening clinical status on antibiotics, his physician appropriately referred him to the ER for advanced evaluation and treatment that could not be offered in an outpatient setting. Upon arrival to the ER, they completed a series of CAT scans that revealed Mr. Frame's final diagnosis of hepatic abscess. In keeping with the guidelines for the management of this type of hepatic abscess, it will require drainage in addition to antibiotics to ensure proper treatment," she said, giving me a curt nod signaling that because I obviously lacked the proper medical deductive reasoning, she would make the patient presentation herself.

Then, turning to the patient, she said, "Nice to meet you, Mr. Frame. We will be speaking with interventional radiology today to coordinate the drainage of your infection. Of course, there is more testing we will need to do as well while we continue your treatment. There will be many more people by to see you—providers from the departments of radiology, infectious disease, gastroenterology, and, of course, the general internal medicine team." She smiled at Mr. Frame the way a person who has everything under her control would, as if to say that nothing could go wrong because a benevolent captain was in command of this ship.

She turned back to me. "Thank you, Dr. Harper. You can go home to rest up for tonight. Make sure to read about how to take a history, the workup of fever of unknown origin, as well as the presentation, evaluation, and treatment of hepatic abscess. Ideally, these are things you would do *before* rounds. Thank you again. I'm sure we all learned a great deal from your presentation."

"Yes, of course, Dr. Jaiswal."

With that, she pivoted on her kitten heels and walked out of the room. One by one, the interns followed, a trail of white coats shuffling behind trying to keep up. One intern tripped on the feet of the one in front of her.

I slinked out of the room, wishing desperately that I could vaporize. That morning, I went home and napped away the day.

I never forgot that encounter. For the entire intern year, I made sure to ask *too many* questions of my patients. After all, it was the clinician's job to get the history. Sure, the patient had to answer questions honestly in order for this to work, but I was the detective, so I needed to know what I was looking for and where to look for it. To the best of my ability, I not only read about the topics I didn't understand, I also read *around* them. I reviewed the history in my head and practiced my assessment and plan, making sure the reasoning led to a logical conclusion. And if I felt that I didn't have all the information from a patient, I went back as many times as required to make sure I got it. Each case was a story, and the story had to make sense.

That was the last time I was unprepared for Dr. Jaiswal's rounds. What's important was that in that very long year, she helped me become a better doctor because I saw the good in her, in the value she placed on meticulous preparation and critical thinking. The other parts, the parts that were derogatory and cruel? I made up my mind to ignore. All of it, the rough and the smooth, was crucial for my development as a doctor. I later realized that even with its excruciating challenges, this intern year prepared me best for the transition from my former life to my life after residency and my divorce.

"Doctor Michele Harper."

My residency program director had called my name, breaking my trance. My final graduation.

I don't remember what I wore to the ceremony, or who

spoke, but I vividly remember how eternally grateful I was for the power to compose myself in the seven seconds it took me to stand and walk to the podium. I claimed my diploma and took the obligatory photos before dissolving into tears. I knew how to compartmentalize—my family dysfunction and my stint in medical school had given me a lot of practice. I didn't have time to grieve for my marriage or for the future my ex-husband and I would never share. I had to pack, move, unpack, coordinate a divorce and the sale of our co-op, and start a new job in a new city, alone. I hadn't even considered the new life part. Thank goodness for that convenient oversight. If I had stopped to consider that for even one moment, I don't know how I would have gotten into the Ford Explorer Dan and I shared—it would be returned to him, as it had been a gift from his family—to make the drive to Philly.

I don't remember much else about my residency graduation because I was striving so hard to let go of that future and struggling to understand that another was already under way. I'd signed a lease for an apartment in one of the upscale buildings in Center City, within walking distance of the hospital where I was to work. The doormen called you by name and asked how your day was going. The elevators ascended silently at warp speed. My thirty-fifth-floor unit was absolutely tranquil, and I had floor-to-ceiling windows that let in waterfalls of light. I hoped these fancy things might fill the void inside me currently inhabited by pain.

For my first night there, I had an air mattress, six boxes

of clothing, two boxes of kitchenware, and my computer. I possessed little else materially. The one item I had taken from our co-op in the South Bronx was a large mirror. I asked Dan to send two items that had been gifts to us: a woven basket from Kenya and a framed photograph of a woman standing at a bus stop in front of the Shepard Fairey Barack Obama HOPE poster. He agreed, but I knew he wouldn't send them, and I couldn't muster the energy to mount any significant protest. They would be just two more parts of a past I had lost.

On one of my first days in the new apartment, I sat for hours on the living room carpet staring out the windows. I could see the signs and façades of neighboring businesses, many of which were owned by my new employer. Unfortunately, the neon sign announcing "Andrew Johnson Hospital" was the biggest during the day and shone brightest during the night. It wasn't reassuring then, and as it turned out, that wouldn't change. Still, I could just make out a corner of the Schuylkill River snaking along the horizon, which offered a calming contrast to the cityscape.

The particulate matter of memory, heavy and unrefined, filled the room. I inhaled it, letting it abrade the back of my throat and sting my eyes. I lifted my chin into peak June sunlight. Closing my eyes, I leaned into the gold, orange, and red behind my eyelids. I was drawn to it, like a plant. I felt my skin baking. I felt the crackle of the heat, but I didn't flinch: I was finally feeling something. I didn't know what existed beyond the window, beyond the door to my apartment. I didn't know myself in this place. I didn't know what I would be. I fancied that all things happened for a reason, so there had to be a reason I had been stripped to my core and was sitting here on a warm carpet, in the blazing reflected light of an unknown city. In a couple of days, I would unpack these boxes, don crisp green scrubs, and go to work. Sometime soon, I'd figure out the rest, but now, I just had to be broken. There wasn't energy for much else.

A cloud breezed by, offering a moment's respite from the heat. Thank the goddess for those windows. For the light. For the silence. Thank the goddess for the view from thirty-five stories up: I didn't yet recognize anything I saw from that height, but it offered a critical distance, a life-saving perspective.

THREE

Baby Doe: Born Perfect

NIGHT SHIFTS ARE ALWAYS inconvenient and much like hangovers: The older you get, the harder they are to recover from. For some, they are a badge of honor; those types sprint them like marathons, race after race, year after year, with the stamina of a long-distance runner. The nocturnists, the hospital-based physicians who are scheduled to work the night shift exclusively, are the strong and brave among us. The goddess forever blesses them because they allow the rest of us to dwell largely in the light.

While night shifts are a brutal subjugation of my natural diurnal instinct—yes, I prefer to conduct my life during the day and sleep at night—I have to admit that sometimes they're a refuge. Sometimes it's nice to leave the distractions of the daytime and let myself be swallowed whole by the night. I don't have to respond to emails, or make phone calls, or schedule meetings, or do much of anything else when I'm working in the emergency room at night. In this way, it's a nice break from my administrative work.

Don't get me wrong, I signed up for admin. It was my habit, my well-worn groove. I wasn't comfortable if I wasn't in a leadership role. It was a routine I leaned into. After all, back in the early 1990s I had started a club I called Future Doctors of America at my high school (although, at the time, I wasn't entirely sure I wouldn't be an architect or an attorney instead), I was student government president my senior year, co-chaired our local branch of the American Medical Women's Association while in medical school, and was a chief resident my final year in residency. Naturally, I thought I wanted to continue in leadership roles in the hospital while I worked as an attending ER physician.

So, here I was, at Philadelphia's Andrew Johnson Hospital, a large teaching institution where I would have to prove myself. I started small, as the director of performance improvement in the emergency department. It was fascinating reviewing cases to investigate potential clinical errors, cases where, for example, a doctor or nurse practitioner (each called a "provider" in health care lingo) had made an inaccurate diagnosis or prescribed suboptimal treatment. These cases were typically referred to me based on grievances about patient care in the emergency department made by physicians in other hospital departments, by the hospital legal department, or by patients. Initially, I enjoyed the detective work involved in uncovering subtle system failures. It quickly became clear to me, however, that no matter how deferentially I approached my colleagues on these matters, they were not thrilled to hear from me. A physician who has made a mistake (a misdiagnosis, a procedural misstep) never wants to hear the doctor in charge of case review ask him, "Remember the case . . . ?" While I had gotten over the need to be liked or feel externally validated sometime before, it was still unpleasant to be received like the in-law you are obligated to speak to at Thanksgiving dinner despite not really wanting to.

But while working nights in the ED, I found all of that melting away. In preparation for those shifts, I take off my administrative hat, close my laptop, and silence my phone. During night tours, I am able to budget time for one morning activity, plus sleep, before heading back to work again. I choose carefully what will occupy this prized morning slot. On a beautiful morning in late summer, I might have my pick of the most succulent blueberries and the most verdant kale at the farmers' market, but I usually head straight to the gym. All the nine-to-fivers are on their way to the office by the time I get there, and anybody who isn't working is still making their first cup of coffee, so I can enjoy the gym in peace—just me and the eighty-year-old man who seems never to leave.

When I'm done, I go home to a cup of Sleepytime tea and the most indulgent nap on the softest, cotton candy pink organic sheets. When else can an adult intentionally sleep the day away and be called responsible for doing so?

Later, at 4:30 p.m., the alarm on my phone will chirp, and it will be time to get up, as my next night shift begins. I'll walk through the hospital doors just before 7 p.m., in time to see the big smile on the face of the doctor at the end of the day shift. Things always start the same way: I consult the "sign-out," a list of the outstanding tasks the day physician couldn't resolve during her time on, and begin digging myself out of a hole. It never matters if the sign-out list contains two items or ten; it always feels like too many given the inevitable backup of patients currently waiting to be seen and the steady influx of new patients arriving over the course of the next twelve hours.

On one particular evening, I was the sole physician in the ED and was sharing the shift with the night nurses Crystal and Deb. It's always a blessing to have a strong and amusing team when you're on nights. When everything is stripped to bare bones, it's a boon to have a sturdy foundation. I notice that the nurse Pam is on, too, and I tell myself that you can't expect everyone on the team to be great. Pam is reasonably intelligent, but her clinical insight is often hampered by a bizarre emotional instability. I couldn't figure out how she'd ended up in emergency medicine, but why she hadn't been fired was obvious: Pam was committed to nights. The committed night crew is untouchable. Hospitals need them to reliably absorb the burden of the shifts other nurses don't want to do.

We chugged along uneventfully until around 1 a.m., at which point we heard an ambulance backing into the ambulance bay. Then EMS rolled in a CHFer (our abbreviation for heart failure patients) puffing away on a portable BiPAP

(bilevel positive airway pressure) machine. A plump
woman dressed in what looked like a housecoat lay
gurney. The nurses established intravenous lines a
formed the woman that they wanted to administer the
cation Lasix into her vein to help her urinate the extr
backing up into her lungs, as the respiratory tech sw
her over to the hospital's BiPAP face mask to help her bı
I leaned over and asked her, in a voice raised just eno
overcome the blowing of the BiPAP machine but not
approximating a yell, "Ms. Yang, how are you feeling?"

She smiled behind the mask as the forced air ma
cheeks flap, then flashed a thumbs-up to let me know sł
improving. Her EKG and physical exam indicated th
heart was stable, so we were on autopilot for now. The
team headed back out the door, and then one of the l
returned to give us a heads-up that we might be getting
diatric code. He said he had been listening to the radi
had heard a call about a baby not breathing and he wan
alert us in case it was coming our way.

"I certainly hope not! Last thing I need in the mid
the night," Pam said, loud enough for all twelve beds i
ER to hear.

My physician assistant had just left, there were si
tients in the ER, one had just been brought in, and
more were in the waiting room, so the news of the
wasn't something I was enthusiastic about either. The
is, there is never a good time for a pediatric code. Whe
adult gets sick, we can reason about how or why. Afte

Grandpa has to die of something. And if Dad binge-drank every week for the past forty years, we're not shocked when his liver fails. If Mom was a diabetic who loved to smoke, we understand when she has a heart attack. Even in cases of seemingly random illnesses, such as breast cancer in a thirty-six-year-old man, while these are painful and difficult to absorb, we can concoct for ourselves a kind of piecemeal comprehension to get through somehow. But when a child is brought in with a critical illness, such as cancer or organ failure, we experience a different kind of suffering. Because we see them as both innocent and invincible—too young to justify the affliction and certainly too perfect to succumb to it—it is that much harder to wrestle with.

I moved on to Mr. Nuñez, in Bed 3, while I awaited Ms. Yang's test results. Depending on her labs, I would admit her to a regular floor bed with heart monitoring, or to the cardiac intensive care unit for her CHF exacerbation. While I assisted the tech in splinting Mr. Nuñez, who had come in with a wrist fracture, the alert came through.

Pediatric code blue. ETA five minutes. Pediatric code blue. ETA five minutes.

I knew it was too much to hope for that we'd be spared.

I asked Crystal to place Mr. Nuñez in a sling and quickly printed his discharge papers. Deb's phone rang. One of the medics was calling with an update—a benefit of having someone on shift who is friends with a local paramedic.

"Doc, neonate not breathing," Deb said when she got off

the phone. "They coded in the field ten minutes, couldn't intubate, but have IV access. They'll be here any minute."

Ms. Yang, the CHF patient, was doing well. A quick look at the computer revealed that her labs were coming back normal. It was likely that she hadn't had a heart attack, just a serious flare-up of her congestive heart failure. I asked the clerk, Wendy, to call the hospitalist, the doctor overseeing the medical admissions for the shift, and put the patient's name in for a bed. We needed to admit her immediately to clear the decks. There was no telling how long a baby code would take.

I took a quick inventory of the status of the remaining patients. Mr. Nuñez was going home. The three waiting room patients had normal vital signs with no life-threatening complaints, so they could wait. Two patients had already been admitted to the hospital and were just waiting for beds to open up. Two more patients were waiting to go to Radiology for CT scans.

"Okay, let's prep the Resuscitation Room," I said, heading there with my crew of nurses. "Crystal, can you please make sure we have suction? Make sure the code cart is at bedside. Let's bring out the neonate tray. And let's lay out the Broselow tape here," I directed. "Who's gonna write?" I asked the crew.

"I will," Pam responded, already wheeling over a bedside table with a code sheet, the document that records a chronology of all resuscitative efforts during a code in hand.

"Excellent. Okay, are the meds there? Ready with the pediatric pads?" I asked.

"Yup," said Mark, the tech, holding up the pads for pediatric defibrillation from the pediatric code cart.

"Let me grab my mask and gloves. Miller and ET tube ready." Then I noticed something. "Wait, there's no Miller zero in the department? All I have is a one. Good to have a zero in case the kid is small," I said as I laid down the Miller laryngoscope, the tool used to open and visualize the airway, and the endotracheal tube, which is inserted into the trachea for ventilation, both at the head of the bed near my right hand.

Mark looked around the code cart, grabbing different trays—to no avail: There wasn't a size zero to be found in the ER.

"Well, then, this will have to work!" I grabbed the Yankauer, the long plastic suctioning tip used in various oral medical procedures, and tested it against my gloved hand. "Suction is good," I said, tucking it under the mattress head. "Ready!"

Then we stood there staring at one another.

The hardest moments are those right before the code arrives, when the air is thick with anticipation of all the terrible things that could happen and we have time to wrestle with each grisly scenario. I secretly preferred it when the EMS team rolled a patient in unannounced. Sure, we would whine and moan because we had to scramble to prepare everything while treating the patient at the same time, but in reality, such a scenario afforded us the opportunity—really, the luxury—of just being in the moment, of doing our job without getting tangled up in the *story* of the job. Most of the time, though, EMS teams have the courtesy to call ahead. So we stood around the stretcher, reminding ourselves to breathe.

"What a shitty thing for a Wednesday night," Pam said.

A cascade of beeps broke the silence. A convenient feature of this resuscitation room, apart from being spacious, was that it offered a clear view of the ambulance entrance. We stood there at attention as the ambulance backed up to the ER, flashing lights that whirled across the bay doors and floors in a dizzying rotation. Then, with a whoosh, two medics swooped in, pushing a small gurney with a tiny patient swathed in white.

"Newborn baby, twelve days old," the first medic reported. "Called for not breathing. Not breathing on scene. No pulse. CPR started. Family is on the way. We didn't get the baby's name; we just got to work. Family can fill in those details when they get here."

"Okay, we'll just register him as Doe, like we always do," Pam interjected.

They parked the gurney next to our stretcher and transferred the baby as one medic continued to ventilate the patient by securing the bag valve mask over his face while squeezing the little chamber of air connected to it in order to deliver oxygen to the baby's lungs.

"How long was the baby down?" I asked.

"We don't know. Parents went in to check on him and found him like this," he responded.

"How long were you coding in the field?"

"Ten minutes at the scene. About six minutes en route. No return of circulation."

"Okay. What did you give?"

"Three rounds of epi. Accu-Chek eighty-two, so no need for glucose. IO left lower extremity. Unable to tube in the field."

As the medic and I talked, Deb was frantically connecting leads from our monitor to the infant. Placing my fingers on the inner aspect of the baby's upper arm, I noted no pulse at the brachial artery. Moving my fingers to the crease at the upper thigh on the same side, I noted no pulse at the femoral artery. Shifting my gaze to the monitor briefly, I saw no shockable rhythm on our monitor. The skin was warm and soft. So smooth—just like a baby's. I listened to the chest to observe that nothing was moving. There was no heartbeat, no sounds of breathing.

"Mark, please start chest compressions," I said, bracing myself and trying to sound calm.

Mark placed what seemed like a giant's fingers on the child's tiny sternum and began to rhythmically press.

"Okay, another dose of epi," I instructed. "Pam, please let me know when it's time for another. Just give a heads-up about the epi at five-minute intervals," I requested. "Can we just confirm that blood sugar? And I'll start intubating."

I looked down at the little boy's face for the first time. Dark eyes that were wide-open. Beautiful brown skin with a bluish cast. If this child had still been alive, he would have borne a strong resemblance to my sister's infant son, Eli. He was the specter of the child I didn't have, the ghost of What Might Have Been. His beauty welled up in my eyes, and I had to blink myself back to reality. This was little angel Doe. At first glance it was impossible to tell if his eyes were black or merely dark from the pupils being fixed and dilated; in either case, there was nothing behind them. His little purple, pouty lips were half-parted where he'd exhaled goodbye long ago. His face was still encircled by the white of the baby blanket that crowned his head. There was no baby here, just a blanket around the body of a departed cherub.

I looked up at Deb. She knew it, too. Everyone around the stretcher knew. We know when a lifeless pod is brought through the door, but we're supposed to make heroic efforts at resuscitation as they do on TV, when the body is already stiff and blue, but the family is not ready; when arms that have lost the current of life fall limp to the side rails. Still, we push several rounds of meds into them, just to document to the family, peer review boards, and the courts what we already know to be true.

I took a deep breath as I positioned the baby boy's tiny head and gently placed the Miller blade between his lips. The blade seemed far too large for his mouth. As I advanced the laryngoscope and lifted it up to expose his vocal cords in order to insert the breathing tube, there was tension at the corners of his lips from the size of the blade. I withdrew, opened his jaw, and advanced again. Again, the blade seemed too big. I didn't want to force it through his mouth.

I couldn't believe what was happening. Shortly after starting this job, I had completed Dr. Rich Levitan's difficult airway course, in which this renowned guru of emergency medicine gave us his pearls of wisdom regarding endotracheal intubation. The chairman of the hospital's emergency department had been kind enough to send any interested faculty members to the lab Rich ran in Baltimore to attend this class. Even before the course, I had never missed a pediatric intubation during my residency. Outside of some anatomic abnormality, children were the easiest to intubate. Because the pediatric airway is shorter and more anterior than in adults, the epiglottis, the landmark we often use to locate the vocal cords for endotracheal intubation, is typically so easily visible that you can see it when kids laugh. Given that you didn't usually need a blade to see their epiglottises, technically speaking, there was nothing to most pediatric intubations. And yet now I couldn't do it.

My heart pounded in my fingertips, and I could feel everyone's eyes on me as I struggled to avoid harming the baby. I knew he was gone, but I couldn't bear the thought of making one tiny cut or scratch on this immaculate little being. I couldn't mar perfection.

Resuscitations can be brutal: Ribs are broken with chest compressions, skin is contused, mouths bloodied, even teeth knocked out, for God's sake. And then, only *rarely*, after all this medically induced trauma, are people electrocuted back from the dead.

I had long been inured to the assaults that medical teams perpetrate on patients for what is considered the greater good—until now, when the thought of rendering the tiniest blemish on the body of this dead infant made my hands seize up.

"Is there a smaller blade? Do we have a Miller zero?" I asked again, muting my panic. It was an absurd question, as I already knew the answer.

The nurses scrambled to search the cart again, but still found nothing. We continued the resuscitation, with me holding the mask over the baby's face, squeezing the bag of oxygen to ventilate the child until an advanced airway could be secured with an endotracheal tube.

"I'm going out to the truck. I'm pretty sure we have a smaller blade, Doc," said one of the medics who had hung back to watch the code and help out if needed.

In seconds, he returned with a Miller 0. As I began again, I thought to myself, This has to be better. Certainly, now I could advance without breaking his little baby jaw. I gently inserted the blade, and *still* it seemed too big. I met resistance right at the tongue. I couldn't stretch the mouth. I couldn't bruise the gums. I couldn't force the blade back and up. Once again I tried, and once again I failed.

"Doc, do you mind if I try?" the same paramedic inquired. I didn't look up. I just stepped aside.

"Pam, what's the time?" I asked.

"Time for another epi, Doc. Ten minutes."

"Okay, please give another," I directed.

I asked the medic if he was ready to try for the tube, and he said yes. "Please hold compressions one moment for intubation," I announced to the crew.

The medic drove the blade between the jaws and cranked forward. The corners of the mouth stretched taut, the skin ripping at both corners, thereby permitting the blade. In the same swoop, the neck craned forward, allowing the passage of a small breathing tube. At the medic's first attempt, the tube was in.

We continued the fruitless attempts at resuscitation for another ten minutes.

It was finally time for the inevitable end to the code (one that could easily have been called soon after the infant's arrival), wherein I pronounced the time of death. The code had, in actuality, ended long before the baby was rolled into the department. The child had died at home. The time I called in the ER would simply be a formality.

I looked around at the team and said, "Guys, this kid is really gone. Does anyone have any further ideas before we call the code?"

"No, Doc. There's nothing else to do," one of the nurses said.

One by one, the members of the team shook their heads.

"Any objections to my calling the code now?" I asked. I got a chorus of "No, Doc."

We took our hands off the baby, the bed, the monitors. I

checked the nonreactive pupils and the chest—no breath sounds, no heartbeat, no life.

"Time of death, one forty-one a.m. Thank you, everyone. Thank you for all the hard work. Is the family here?"

"They're out in the waiting room," Pam said.

I sighed and shook my head. "Okay, so who's gonna go out with me?" I threw off my gloves and mask as I exited the room.

Deb stepped forward and rubbed my arm, signaling support for my efforts and that she'd be the one. The doctor typically doesn't speak with the family alone. They often need more time and support than any ER physician is able to give between patients, so usually a nurse or hospital staff member comes along for the discussion. During the day, it's nice when a chaplain or social worker is available.

Now we were heading into the hardest part of the code, the part that had no algorithm, no script, the raw part that never feels good.

"By the way," I said, as I stopped and turned back to the group. "Did we ever get a name on the baby?"

Wendy got up from her desk, which was situated at the front of the ER between the Resuscitation Room and front entrance just kitty-corner to both, to answer, "Baby Christopher Tally. I verified it with the parents. Everyone's out there. Want me to go get them? You could take them to the back office to talk."

"Thanks, Wendy. It's okay. I'm going out." Then Deb and I headed to the waiting room.

A crowd of people filled the room. A person I figured was the mother was wringing her hands, a trail of tears blazing down her cheeks. She and a man I assumed to be the father were standing near the door, holding each other up. His eyes were red and puffy.

Parents know. They know the way we know life is gone as the gurney is rolled through the ambulance doors. Parents know because these angels whisper their last words in their ears and butterfly-kiss them good-bye. The others in the waiting room were sitting or pacing, both fearful and hopeful in their anxiety.

"Hello, I'm Dr. Harper," I said. "Are you the Tally family?" They all stiffened.

The mother's eyes were clouded with grief. "Yes," she whispered.

"Please come with me," I said.

An older woman among them stood and told everyone but the parents to stay in the waiting room. She was authoritative, an upright and strong presence. I figured she was the grandmother. The husband supported the mother on the right side and the grandmother on the left as they ushered Mom through the waiting room doors and into the front of the ER. The curtains in front of the Resuscitation Room, which was just feet away, had been drawn so they could not yet view the scene.

"Would you like to come with me to the room right over there where we can sit?" I asked.

"No," the mother whimpered. "Please, please, just tell me now," she implored.

If she hadn't been held up on both sides, she would have tumbled to the floor. She began to wail and sway.

"Jessica, please, please let the doctor talk," her mother said as she stroked her daughter's hair.

Deb asked again, "Are you sure you all don't want seats?"

"Nooooooo, teeeelllll meeee!" the mother shrieked as she clutched her chest.

Her mother embraced her and turned toward me. "I'm sorry. It's okay. You can tell us."

"I'm very sorr—" I began, but before I could finish the word, the mother fell to the floor.

She had already known, but the words were irrevocable confirmation. The father collapsed as well and lay embracing her on the floor. The grandmother gasped, clasping her left hand over her mouth and holding her right hand to her breast. She stood tall. Her watery eyes held fast.

There was no space between the mother's cries for me to say anything, no space for words.

I could not share the thoughts that were circling in my mind: There was no space in their grief. I couldn't tell them, *I'm very sorry you lost your angel baby. I'm very sorry he died while you were sleeping and you didn't get to say good-bye. I'm so sorry that he was already dead when the EMS team arrived and that despite that thirty-five minutes of squeezing his tiny heart and pumping it full of enough drugs to jump-start a car, we couldn't summon him back to life. I'm sorry I couldn't intubate your baby. I'm sorry. It's just that when I propped up his tiny head and inserted the laryngoscope blade, I felt I was hurting him. I'm sorry that the last thing his little corpse experienced was prodding and poking and pressing and tearing. I'm sorry that your beautiful boy is gone. I'm sorry that I can't tell you why, and I'm sorry I can't make it hurt any less.*

"I'm so sorry. I'm so very sorry," I said into the space. Everyone else in the front end of the department was silent. The only sound was the parents' wailing and a distant shuffling in the back of the ER. Then the mother tore back the curtain and ran to her baby, spilling once again to the tile beneath her feet. The father was not far behind, crying and pacing and barely able to support his own weight against gravity.

"How did this happen? Why did this happen? He was perfect! He was perfect! Nothing was wrong! Nothing was wrong," the mother yelled up to the sky, invisible beyond the hospital ceiling.

The grandmother walked to her side and collected her daughter from the floor.

A call came in at Wendy's desk: the mother's obstetrician phoning our department. Wendy answered it and walked over to the mother.

"Mrs. Tally, a Dr. Thomas is on the phone for you. Would you like to take it?"

"Yes, yes," the woman managed to say, and followed Wendy to the phone. She grabbed the receiver in her right hand, cradling her head in her left hand as she braced herself against the section of the counter encircling the doctors' and nurses' station that was in front of Wendy. "Dr. Thomas! I don't know what happened! I don't know what happened!" Then she listened for a moment and responded. "I know, I know . . . I know . . ." She dissolved into sobs. "There was nothing wrong the whole nine months . . . I know . . . I know . . ."

The grandmother had just returned from the waiting room, where she had gone to notify the rest of the family. I walked over to her.

"I'm very sorry," I told her. "Do you have any questions? Is there anything we can do for you?"

"Do you know what happened?" she asked.

"I know that when EMS responded to the nine-one-one call, Christopher was not breathing and his heart was not beating. He was not alive at that time. EMS worked really hard to try to bring him back. They gave him medicine to try to start his heart again and make him breathe, but they were not able to bring him back. When he arrived here his heart was not beating and he was not breathing. He was not alive. We continued these efforts when he arrived, but we were not able to bring him back, either."

She stood facing me, heartbroken, silent with grief.

"Do you know if he was sick at all? Were there any problems with the pregnancy or delivery or after?" I asked her.

"No. It was tough for them to get pregnant, but when they finally did, everything went well. She was never sick.

The delivery went well. They were out of the hospital in two days. The baby had a perfect checkup visit. Everything was perfect." She stared at me. "How does this happen?" she asked, shaking her head.

I took a breath. "It's so hard to say. Sometimes it's an underlying medical problem a baby is born with. It's nobody's fault. It's just one of those things in nature. Other times, we never have any diagnosable reason for why it happens. Again, I am truly sorry."

"Thank you, thank you," she said, before lowering her head and walking back over to her daughter.

Dr. Thomas asked to speak to me. I took the phone and, at the request of the family, informed her of what had happened. She told me the story of the difficult conception. She recounted how happy the parents had been to be pregnant. They were such a cute, hardworking couple, she said. She told me she had known the young woman since she was sixteen years old, and now here it was, sixteen years later, and she was delivering her first baby. Everything had gone like clockwork. Her voice cracked as we said our good-byes and acknowledged that it had been a very hard night.

As I ticked the pertinent boxes on the death note and hospital chart, my mind began to wander, but I had to keep redirecting my energy to the work. I sent off an email to the medical director requesting smaller pediatric blades in the event of future neonatal codes, one more discussion point for the next staff meeting. I heard Pam muttering to the tech that

I should have been able to intubate the child, that there had been no equipment problem; the issue had been me. The tech responded that it didn't really make a difference, since there had been no bringing the dead infant back to life. I heard Deb say that we really should have proper pediatric equipment and that Pam shouldn't be criticizing me so harshly.

I spoke to the medical examiner on call, then notified Organ Donation that this, like any neonatal death, would be a medical examiner case, so not a candidate for organ dona-tion. Ultimately, the family left, and Baby Tally was wrapped snugly in his white blanket and rolled away to the morgue.

One by one, the hours passed.

Finally, my shift ended and I found myself at home as the sun rose. I drank a glass of red wine, chased it with chamo-mile tea and a Benadryl, and fell into a shallow sleep. Hours later, I awoke feeling heavy and with one thought: I had failed the baby. It was two hours before night shift number two this week.

I knew that my mother would be off work by now. I picked up the phone to call, to tell her of my failure while I prepared my dinner. I stood over my new yellow soup pot from Williams-Sonoma—the pot was part of my strategy to buy fancy cookware to encourage me to cook, to get on with life. Much like the monthly auto-renew membership to my yoga studio, this strategy, of investing financially in some-thing that would force me to participate in life, always worked. I couldn't stare at my pricey pots, pans, and high-speed blender without feeling sufficient guilt over not making use of them regularly.

As the soup simmered, I choked on a flood of tears. In that moment, I realized that in all my years of training, I had never really cried. During my residency, when people were brought into the emergency room beaten and stabbed and later died in my arms, I didn't cry. At family conferences, when I had to inform wives that I'd had to put their husbands on ventilators and had no idea whether those men would ever breathe on their own again, there were no tears.

And when I had been a desperate girl, a child without a childhood, praying to the crescent moon at midnight that my family might survive, that I might survive, I didn't cry. The pain might have scorched my throat, my eyes might have misted up, but I never truly let myself feel the burn, never lowered the floodgates. My divorce only months before had shattered me in ways I had never imagined, but even then, I hadn't fully allowed myself the luxury of a stream of tears. There wasn't time. I had to get through it; I had to push past it to survive and excel. Now here, after graduations, after my divorce, between night shifts, between the cracks in the crumbling stories I had told myself of what my life should look like by now, there was an opening for reflection.

The truth was I had never cared about "marriage." I was never a girl who thought there was anything special about the title of "wife." Both its historical roots (women used as property) and the state defining legitimate versus illegitimate love to bolster both the patriarchy and the heteronormativity on which it depends had stained the institution in my eyes. Instead, I valued a spiritual union, which is something that can never be bestowed by anybody besides the two souls in the relationship. Sure, traditional marriage made sense from a business perspective, if the conditions of that business were best served by such a contract.

When I was young, I didn't dream of being a mother. Most people I knew of chose a partner with the same level of meaningful intention as Ken marrying Barbie, then reproduced reflexively like cattle, so, in my estimation, the mere acts of coupling and multiplying never conferred any singular importance or achievement to neither humans nor the one-celled organisms who can do this too. I figured motherhood would happen for me one day in the future, when I got around to it. It wasn't something I needed to do, but I took for granted that I would. I suppose I took it for granted in the same way I assumed that I would encounter the partner with whom it would make sense to share my life—settling was not an option.

I stood stirring my soup of the day, a rustic chicken stew with quinoa, chickpeas, and a selection of veggies, allowing rivers of salt to flow down my face. With each turn of the spoon in the pot, I remembered what it was I actually missed: a healthy, soulful connection to another person. And now that the option of having a family seemed to have evaporated,

I grieved that I'd lost the chance to do childhood and spiritual marriage right, the way I had never known them for myself.

During our call that day, I told my mother about Baby Tally. I recounted how he had looked like Eli and the baby I didn't have. I told her that this new city was far lonelier than I had ever imagined possible. But worst of all was that I might never get to raise a child the way a child should be raised, to provide her with the love and shelter she deserved.

My mother responded reflexively the way many mothers feel they have to. She told me that the baby's death hadn't been my fault, that none of it was my fault. She ended with a statement as certain as fact that of course I would have the family I wanted one day. She spoke as if time weren't a factor, as if the future held limitless possibilities for me—whatever I wanted.

But I knew better. I knew that days morph into years, which turn into decades that don't promise particular outcomes. In the same way, no matter how "perfect," a soul can take its leave from earth in twelve days or twelve years without so much as a hint.

It's human nature to want to bind ourselves to the parts of life we hold dear whether those parts are actual people, events, items, or dreams. We want to fasten them to us so they're safe and near us forever. But this type of binding frays and tears until, even when we fight the awareness, we're forced to see how illusory the reliance on permanence is. What we have, in all its glory, to hug and hold, to caress and learn, to feel and grow, is simply right here and right now. If we are lucky, the bond holds in the moment—and the experience of it shines and breathes and expands. Then our story can change in an instant, and we may never be given the gift of *why*.

I didn't have an answer. Baby Tally's family didn't have an answer. We had all been broken in that moment—broken open by shock and grief and anger and fear. I didn't know how or when, but this opening could lead to healing. After all, only an empty vessel can be filled by grace; but to get there, we had to help each other rise while we shed the same tears. We had to get up and start again.

FOUR

Erik: Violent Behavior Alert

FOUR A.M. IS OFTEN a magic hour. In emergency departments all over, chances are there will be a lull in, and respite from, the action at around this time. The main overhead lights of the ER will still be turned down to accommodate patient rest for a couple more hours before the change in shift. It's a time when the doctor on duty can catch up on paperwork or other tasks, and maybe even steal a moment, as she sits at her desk, to watch the barest beginning of sunrise glistening through the windowpane. She squints as her eyes adjust to daylight and longs for the moment when she can walk out of the hospital inspirited by the light of a brand-new day. And for a couple of hours, she is reminded that she, too, is a diurnal human being.

In several hours, at 7 a.m., before I'm free to get in my car and drive home, I will take my place around a large walnut table with six nurses and two other physicians for the code meeting, where we will review issues regarding any medical resuscitations performed in the hospital. Together we will pore over the long code sheet, finding where the word *atropine* was written during a patient resuscitation on the telemetry unit last week. "The exact location of this wording is critical to saving lives," said no one ever who actually saves lives. Nevertheless, after twenty minutes of our discussing the word's location, I will endure a similarly inconsequential discussion about whether to move the space on the code sheet for "fingerstick glucose." During a 4 a.m. lull on the night shift, I prepare my thoughts on these matters, thoughts that boil down to one question: Why are we meeting about this?

Tomorrow I will get the notification, the phone call or email that I hope will announce the promotion that will deliver me from being merely an attendee at such meetings to being the chair. Just under two years into the relatively minor administrative positions of director of departmental performance improvement and then ED assistant medical director, I was bored. The hospital had just created a new position for an administrator to oversee quality on a larger scale throughout its operations. It was a job I wanted and knew I would be good at. My ED chair couldn't promote me any further within the department—the existing directors weren't going to be leaving or dying anytime soon—and therefore supported me in pursuing the position.

I had assessed there might be more meaning for me, more potential for me to make an impact, when I was in charge of something. I knew that when I prescribed rest, ice, compression, and elevation to a patient with an ankle sprain or explained to a patient with tooth pain that there wasn't an abscess or dental emergency, but that it was critical for her to follow up with a dentist for a detailed exam—when I did these things, I knew that these patients could hear me and that there was the potential for something important to be accomplished. I also knew that in no part of my medical training had I dreamed of spending hours contemplating how best to make sure blood cultures were drawn within four hours of a patient's being admitted to a regular hospital floor with community-acquired pneumonia. Frankly, it felt unfair having to spend so much of my life as a physician ruminating over minutiae that didn't actually improve people's lives. There had to be ways for me to climb this administrative ladder meaningfully. I'd find out tomorrow.

Since graduating from my residency a couple of years before, I'd grown increasingly jaded and restless, and was not sure that working at an administrative level in a hospital was even what I wanted to do anymore. Yoga was helping me to cope and clarify. Gym workouts were helping, too, as was expanding my social circle. I had succumbed to peer pressure to join the online dating scene, in an effort to "get back out there"—this, specifically, did not help—but my entry into that world had been hesitant at best. It had nothing to do with fear; for the first time in my life, I was beginning to feel that I had found a certain comfort in my own skin.

The beautiful and unexpected gift of my thirties was that

I liked myself no matter the bumps or blemishes, or the raucous laughter that erupted into snorts under the right circumstances, or the smelly farts from the yummy lentil soup I made (so delicious, but I learned to enjoy it sparingly). My aversion to online dating had nothing to do with the vulnerability of putting oneself on exhibition to thousands of strangers. To the contrary, I'd always found it fascinating to share a conversation with someone entirely unknown. I firmly believe that any interaction can be meaningful, even if only a brief exchange. No, I wasn't afraid of online dating. I just wasn't sold on its effectiveness. Yes, I was well aware of the compelling arguments of two friends who had met their current husbands online. (The same two friends later told me, independent of each other, that they would get divorced if only they had the energy to be single again, but they preferred to settle for an unhappy marriage as a means to ensure they could have a child before the "advanced maternal age" of thirty-five.) Given that I didn't need "practice" in dating, the notion of wading through hundreds of online profiles seemed to be merely a way to settle for Mr. I-Guess-I'll-Give-Up-Give-In-and-Make-It-Work-Somehow in a more time-efficient manner.

I knew also that, for me, a relationship could be only with a man with whom I recognized a soul connection. None of me feels that this type of link can be jury-rigged by any virtual algorithm, no matter how inventive Silicon Valley considers its calculations.

Still, eventually, I had relented, but I made sure to deploy the excuse of my tricky emergency medicine schedule to keep my involvement in the process (what amounted to a couple of months) only tangential. There was Rick, who had clearly posted a photo from twenty years prior and had a penchant for discussing beer and golf exclusively. (I disliked both only a little less than I disliked him.) There was Doug, who repeatedly reminded me that he was an attorney, no matter the topic of conversation; yet, when I finally bit and asked where he practiced law, he gave a verbose answer about the many ways one can be an attorney and not actually practice law, weaving in a discussion of his entrepreneurial interests. I felt my eyes glaze over as I listened to the man lie about his identity. And I can't leave out Frank, who had obviously posted someone else's photo entirely. He rambled on about his divorce from seven years before; how he had no hobbies, few friends, and spent all his free time co-parenting a teenager who appeared not to want to spend any time with him. It was for all these reasons that he figured he'd meet a companion through online dating. I politely finished my drink, stating, "Ugh, so sorry. I'd better rush home. I have to get to the ER tomorrow. I know it's only six-fifteen p.m. now, but my morning shift starts *super early* . . . No, please. You stay and enjoy. I'm safe to walk home, and I walk pretty fast, so I don't want to be rude." I pushed my chair back to wriggle myself free from the booth. "Have a beautiful night," I added, already halfway to the door.

Frank was the last. It was my experience with Frank that

made it clear he *should* be the last. There were no regrets. And thankfully, all of them got away.

I planned to use the 4 a.m. lull to *avoid* responding to the latest two date requests and instead get the code meeting preparation out of the way. Of course, in an ER, downtime is never guaranteed at any hour. Just two weeks earlier, I had worked nonstop straight through the night. I hurried to send home the drunk who had come in ten hours earlier and finally gotten a purchase on sobriety. The CT report on my patient in Room 9 had confirmed appendicitis, so Surgery was called to claim its final patient of the shift. And I had to sew up a facial laceration on an elderly man before admitting a middle-aged woman with multiple rib fractures who had taken a spill down a flight of stairs during a seizure. The stable but hypotensive patient would certainly have to be seen by the next doctor, who was already fourteen minutes late for her shift—but who's counting?

But on this night, a chilly Wednesday in November, the magic hour was holding: At 3:30 a.m., my last patient in the department, a fifty-year-old man complaining of "itchy feet for three months," was well on his way to being cured. There was no rash or infection, just a man who needed lotion. The pharmacist on duty was willing to oblige by sending over a tube of generic moisturizer for the patient to take home to commence the healing, and I could finally sit down at the computer to scroll through my queue on the electronic medical record tracking board to ensure that all my medical notes and orders had been signed. But first I would grab some coffee—I was so tired that my bones ached. Four a.m. tired is nothing like being sore from yoga class or a hard run; it's a deeper throb, a psychic ache.

Here is the blessing and the curse of the 4 a.m. downtime. When everything goes quiet—the techs running back and forth; the patients requesting Percocet, ice, and turkey sandwiches; the nurses asking you to enter all your verbal orders from last night into the computer; a physician on call for a specialty service asking if the consult you placed from the ER is really an emergency or could wait until tomorrow or, better yet, until whatever month a clinic appointment could be made for the patient in question—the inner voice swells until it becomes an existential nudge. Why am I here? What am I *really* doing? What's my purpose?

But who has the energy to navigate this conversation at 4 a.m.?

Yup, it was a good time to get coffee.

Just as I had pushed my chair away from the desk, my screen flashed blue, the color code that told me a new patient had arrived. The magic hour evaporated, and what came up in the complaint tab completely dispelled any charms 4 a.m. usually held: "Hemorrhoid."

The nurses had triaged the patient, Mr. Erik Samuels, with an "emergency severity index" of 4—given that the scale of patient urgency goes, in descending order of severity, from 1 through 5, only a 5 was less critical. So, I wouldn't need to rush. I scrolled through the chart to make sure I didn't miss anything. (Five years later, my memories of rounds with Dr. Jaiswal were still with me.) The patient didn't have a fever, and his other vitals were insignificant: blood pressure 145/86, heart rate 76, respiratory rate 16, saturating 100 percent on room air. I skimmed his electronic medical record. He had a history of hemorrhoids, which each time appeared to have been treated appropriately with a brief course of steroid cream. He also had a history of an inguinal (groin) hernia. Five years before, he had been seen in the hospital's outpatient surgery clinic but had declined any surgical intervention, and then had never returned to that clinic again. It didn't appear to be anything serious.

But then I saw it: A yellow flag appeared on one of the patient's earlier notes, from three years before: "Violent Behavior Alert."

We deal with all kinds of threatening behavior in the ER. By federal law, we are required to evaluate anyone, at any time, with any ailment. For many people, the ER is the only place they can go, particularly those without medical insurance. But it's not the uninsured who use the emergency department the most; it's the insured.

A 2011 survey by the Centers for Disease Control and Prevention explored the reasons the insured find themselves in the ER. Often it is because they feel their health needs aren't being met by their primary care provider; perhaps their doctor doesn't respond quickly enough to their phone call, email, or text. Even when a patient is able to reach their physician to schedule an appointment, they may feel they are simply too sick to wait for the appointment. So, when patients arrive at the ER, they may be delirious from infection or psychotic from a chemical imbalance; they may simply be belligerent drunks, or so entitled from unchecked privilege that even polite questioning causes them to blow a fuse. Whatever the case, it pays to be extremely cautious in the ER.

Actual statistics on violent incidents in emergency departments are sparse; only a small number of dedicated studies have been done. The more pressing issue is that these incidents go largely underreported. The reasons for this are manifold. Many health care providers feel that nothing is done when reports are made, which effectively diminishes the impetus to disclose assaults. Others, fearing they could face scrutiny or blame for not having prevented the violence, become habituated to it: It simply becomes part of the job.

According to the 2003–2007 Workplace Safety Survey by the U.S. Bureau of Labor Statistics, workers in health care and social services are five times more likely to be victims of a nonfatal assault than average workers in all other industries combined. A 2009 Emergency Nurses Association study showed that 20 percent of respondents had been physically assaulted at work more than twenty times in the past three years.

Many television programs don't depict hospital departments accurately. No, the ER staffs are not Hollywood beautiful—you won't find us in the pages of *Vogue* or *GQ*, and we're not all sleeping with one another (I've worked in only one hospital like that)—and given the size of your average American, it turns out it would be extremely difficult to create an emergency airway using a steak knife, a straw, and a bit of twine. But TV does get one part of ER life right: Medical personnel in hospitals are often attacked by the patients they're trying to help. In the most horrifying instances, people walk into hospitals and clinics with guns to murder providers who save lives. Anything can and does happen.

Once I saw the yellow flag on Mr. Samuels's file, I took a deep breath and clicked on the alert note:

Patient grabbed the left breast of female physician while she was performing an incision and drainage on his neck abscess. When it happened, the female physician put down her instrument and left the patient room. The procedure was completed by a male physician.

The rest of the chart read like any other for an abscess treatment, recommending that the patient return in two days for a wound check.

Hot bile constricted the back of my throat, and my face flushed. I didn't know what bothered me most: the patient having committed sexual assault, the offhand manner in which the attack was described, or the fact that the patient was instructed to return to the ER for routine care after he had perpetrated a crime against one of our providers.

Yes, this patient would wait. He would wait while I pushed my chair back, stood up, walked to the break room, poured myself a cup of coffee, went to the restroom, and finished some notes. He would wait until I was done with *everything.* In the comment section next to the patient's name, I typed in "History of assault on staff," and then called the triage nurse to request that he assign Mr. Samuels to one of the male nurses.

"Sure thing. He just has some swelling on his bottom," the nurse responded.

I stood up, secretly hoping that the coffee pot would be empty and I'd have to beg someone to teach me how to brew a new pot. Then I'd wait, drip by drip, until it was ready.

As I turned the corner to head to the staff kitchen, I heard someone shuffling back to Room 7, where Mr. Samuels had been assigned. I heard the dragging of feet and a groan of pain. With my stainless-steel mug in hand, I continued past the sounds to the kitchen.

There are plenty of occupations in which employees have no choice but to deal with anyone who shows up: restaurant server, flight attendant, shoe salesperson, hair stylist. Emergency medicine is the same. But before I became a doctor, I had always assumed there would be less violence and more civility in medicine. We train for a minimum of seven years and spend countless sleepless nights restarting hearts and resetting bones, and yet, now that I was practicing, I knew that we in the ER were no different from those working in service industries. We aren't spared from rude or belligerent patients. We are punched, kicked, called "cunt," and even shot at—none of which should ever happen to anyone in any line of work, but it does. And as doctors, we are exposed to this violence by the very people the law mandates us to treat.

As a resident, I had trained and lived in the South Bronx. Mercy Hospital, one of the busiest hospitals in the country, had good reason to have an in-house police precinct complete with a jail cell. Given the prevalence of violent crime in that part of New York City, and the fact that Mercy was one of the highest-volume trauma centers in the country, people assumed we were under constant threat, but that was not my experience. It's true that we were in the trenches as community members, standing side by side with the South Bronx residents. We knew the police officers, firefighters, and EMTs by their first names. They'd often send the ER staff donuts after we'd helped them unload the fourth gunshot wound, second cardiac arrest, or first pediatric stabbing of the day. We at Mercy might not have had the newest equipment and our scrubs might not have been handsomely monogrammed, but we showed up every day (many of us fueled by the strong and delicious Cuban coffee from the bodega across the street) to take care of as many patients as humanly possible. The faster we worked, the more patients arrived; the more patients, the sicker they seemed to be. If we began a 7 a.m. shift by attending to the twenty-five patients still in the waiting room from 10 p.m. the night before, that simply meant it was a regular Tuesday.

I once treated a patient for a minor GSW to his leg. He was a drug dealer in the neighborhood and, gauging from the substantial roll of money in his pocket, successful in his chosen field. At the end of my shift, he beckoned me over.

"Don't worry about anything around here, Doc. I got

you," he told me—and he meant it. In that way, we were a team. So, I was never physically harmed in the South Bronx.

It wasn't until afterward, when I was working one day at Andrew Johnson's smaller community hospital location, in South Philadelphia, that I encountered my first violent patient, a young man whose mother had brought him in heavily intoxicated. (Although, at twenty-nine, he was technically an adult, in this neighborhood it was a cultural norm for grown men to come to the ER accompanied by their mothers.)

That evening had been peaceful until he was rolled into the department vomiting. The two night nurses who were planning Girl Scout events for their daughters and the evening clerk who was surfing the Web stopped what they were doing to register and triage the new arrival. The patient was deposited in the room kitty-corner to the doctors' station. After safely dumping her son off for the ER staff to deal with, the young man's mother left, and the triage nurse kept his room dark to encourage him to sleep off his intoxication. His was a simple case: I would examine him, prescribe medicine for nausea as well as intravenous hydration, and discharge him back to his parents in the morning. He likely needed none of these treatments; routine intoxication is typically best "treated" by simply kneeling in front of a toilet bowl. But because the young man had been brought to the hospital, we were obligated to provide the medical show the family expected.

"Sir, may I examine you?" I asked.

"Suuuurrrree," he slurred as he moaned and clutched his stomach. He seemed well enough and cooperative.

I told him I would examine him quickly and then the nurse would give him medication for his vomiting. He leaned forward; his lungs were clear. He slumped back; the heart sounds were normal.

"Okay, now open your eyes."

I was inspecting his pupils with the otoscope—the ophthalmoscope head was missing, but really, any light source would have done the trick—when, out of nowhere, a fist came careening toward my face. There was no context to his violence in that moment. There was no good reason and no appropriate justification for it. Being drunk never changes a person, but it does grant their shadow selves free rein to step forward.

I heard my glasses fall to the floor and then slide across the linoleum. In the half-lit room, I saw nothing but a smear of the patient's blond hair and pink skin. As my head jerked, I sensed movement, but I didn't know if it was him or if I was simply readying myself for the next blow. In that same second, I reflexively flung my right arm forward with every ounce of force I could muster, the otoscope still in hand. When it made contact, I heard a crack and a thud as the patient's body reeled back onto the stretcher.

Without my glasses, I was essentially blind—I don't mean blind in the way of needing reading glasses for the morning paper, but blind like I couldn't get to the sidewalk without a walking stick or a guide dog. I knelt carefully to pat down the floor, and luckily my hand reached my glasses, which were right against a cabinet, still intact. I pushed them on and stood. The patient was still lying on the stretcher, his eyes closed. He was breathing, and I didn't see any blood. But I did see a small, red circular impression in the middle of his forehead where the otoscope head had made contact.

At that point, the nurses and the other attending physician had rushed into the room to see if I was all right.

The other attending on shift was Dr. Crist, a six-foot-four retired military man with a voice as big as his stature. He surveyed the scene.

"Well, we'd better add a head CT to his orders," he said.

He continued that he would assume care of the patient, and in his clear, understated way, he declared, "There's no fucking way we should come to work for this shit. These idiots coming in here thinking they can do whatever the hell they want to! Who gives a shit if he's drunk? He's just a lowlife. Why the fuck do these people bring in their shit family so we can take care of them?!"

I just stood there, my face throbbing. I couldn't answer Dr. Crist's questions. They'd been rhetorical, anyway. I appreciated his expressions of rage; my own anger was too choked up in my chest and bound with shame. I didn't know then the exact source of the shame, but I knew what I felt: I was ashamed that a man had struck me in the face; that the blow had left purple welts on my nose and cheek that hurt when I put my glasses back on; I was ashamed that I couldn't scream at the patient or pummel him the way I believe a man who harms a woman deserves to be pummeled. Maybe most of all, I was ashamed that I had been made to feel so weak in my position of supposed power. I was a grown-up now, a doctor, not a child witnessing my father's violence at home.

Big Hector, a nurse whose nickname describes him perfectly, asked if I was okay. The other techs and nurses did, too. They called Security as well. My interaction with the Philadelphia police was brief. An officer took my statement, and we completed the necessary paperwork for the department so that the patient would be banned from care in our hospital system. I declined to press charges, given that it would require a lot of my time to do so and because while I was sure the man's violence had had nothing to do with his inebriation—violence never does—I had doubts about whether the charges would stick in a man with a documented history of intoxication.

Because the incident happened at the end of my shift, I could go right home, something I badly needed to do. When I got to my apartment, I took a naproxen and went to bed with the conviction that I would not dream about what had just taken place.

And now, almost two years later, I was faced with another yellow alert, another reminder of how little power we physicians actually have. Despite my efforts, I couldn't stop thinking about the physician who'd been assaulted by this patient I was about to see. I had tremendous respect for this doctor I'd never met, for the restraint it must have taken for her, after being violated, to calmly put down her scalpel and walk away. I would like to think I would have done the same. I suppose I had, with my inebriated patient—doing just enough to ensure my safety, and then leaving. After all, it was about survival, not retribution. She was lucky she hadn't accidentally killed her assailant when he groped her. But if that had been her reflexive response when under attack, she would have been in the right. It infuriated me that in the world of medicine, a female health care provider could be attacked without consequence, without any means of redress. It was as if patients were permitted such assaults. Why was it that the woman must quietly walk away while the aggressor is allowed to return to the emergency department at any time with the expectation of being serviced?

I stood there in the staff lounge wishing it were easier to be human, wishing we could shed our binary views around gender and power, views that have never served humanity well. I longed for our society to move closer to a harmony where the yellow alerts would fade away so that when I clicked on a patient's history, I would see just another gray computer screen.

It turned out there was coffee in the break room. I touched the side of the pot to find it was still hot. I poured some into my cup and added cream and sugar to the grainy brown brew, thin and watery and likely at least five hours old. In any other circumstances, it would have been unpalatable, but toward the end of a night shift, it was ambrosial. I inhaled—caffeine and a hint of motor oil—and took the first sacred sip.

Now I was prepared for the patient I had no choice but to see.

It was true that I didn't know him at all, so was it fair to judge? I had to admit that there might have been extenuating circumstances to explain this patient's degeneracy—after all, I knew nothing more than what had come up in the notes. Maybe he had been abused as a child. It is not uncommon for boys who are abused to become abusers themselves. It is *never* a justification, of course, but it is an eventuality that deserves compassion. (For all I knew, he had gotten therapy since the assault and was now a fund-raiser for the Rape, Abuse, and Incest National Network. It was a long shot, but it was possible.) It still felt appropriate to make the patient wait, but I knew that there would eventually be other patients to see after him, and it wouldn't be right to delay their care.

I had squandered six minutes, and there was still only one patient in the ER. I grabbed the male nurse who'd been assigned to the patient, Mike, and we headed over to his room.

On the way, Mike grunted under his breath, "I can't believe this guy is allowed to come back here. It's shameful."

I half-smiled at him in solidarity.

The curtain to the room was ajar, revealing a wiry white man lying uncomfortably on the stretcher. His full head of dark hair made him look much younger than he was: His chart said fifty-one. There was no sheet on the bed and no blanket. The man was tall, and naked except for the thin white hospital gown embellished with navy blue geometric shapes. He seemed not to notice or care that as he lay on the stretcher, writhing from side to side, his gown splayed open revealing his bare backside. Mike stood on one side of the room, and I stood next to him and leaned against the supply cart; I needed this bracing as well as the distance. Mike and I stared at the patient as he flopped around like a fish on a hook.

I sighed. Making sure to convey that I was a distant authority figure, I said, "Mr. Samuels, I'm Dr. Harper. What brings you in today?" showing a little less enthusiasm than I might have displayed when asking if he had a paper clip I could borrow.

"The pain, the pain," he moaned. "It happened again!"

"And what might that be, sir?"

"The hernia," he whispered in anguish.

I recalled the triage note in the record. "Hernia? You didn't come in for a hemorrhoid?"

"Well, I don't know what it is. There's something swollen in my groin. It just started today, and I can't take it."

He was curled in the fetal position, his knees bent to his chest. As he spoke, he buried his face in his hands.

"Okay," I said. "Let's take a look at this hernia. Lie on your back."

He tried to relax his legs and attempted to pry them apart. Mike and I regarded him coolly. We didn't move as we waited for him to adjust and calm himself. When he was more still, I walked toward him. His fists were clenched around waves of pain, and his toes twitched with the throbbing. I began to raise his gown and told him to straighten his legs. His arms started to flex up and move toward me. I quickly dropped the edge of his gown and leaned back.

"Put your arms down," I commanded. "Keep your arms down by your sides. Stay still. Straighten your legs."

His thighs were tense as I tapped the side of his right leg. "Okay, open up."

His legs stayed clamped.

I didn't attempt to hide my annoyance. "Sir, would you like to be examined or not?" I continued, already knowing the answer. "The only way I can do that is if you show me the area that is bothering you."

I could sense Mike rolling his eyes, but I was too close to the patient to do anything more than grimace.

The patient lifted his gown and spread his legs enough to reveal a large, firm swelling extending from his right groin to his left scrotum, which was stretched to the size of an eggplant. The skin was so taut that it glistened. Still cautious, but focused, I reached out to palpate his scrotum; I couldn't identify any anatomic landmark. I tried to follow what I imagined might be a thick cordlike swelling down the inguinal canal, but all I could really discern was a balloon of exquisitely tender human flesh. What should I push back into place and where? What was intestine and what was testicle? Was there a perforation or dead bowel? An infection?

I turned to Mike, who had already started to grab supplies.

Our faces softened. This was a surgical emergency. Yes, the man was likely an awful human being, but his pain was real.

"Sir, we will need to put in an IV and check some blood work. We will also need to perform a CAT scan to see what exactly is going on with your hernia. You are right that there is a serious problem here. I have to find out if it's infected and how it is stuck. I will also call a surgeon because you will certainly need an operation to fix this. While all this is going on, we'll make sure you're comfortable. We'll give you pain medication right away."

He looked up at me and nodded. "Thank you, ma'am. Thank you, Doctor."

His eyes were a tremulous, pale gray. I didn't remember the name of the female physician he had assaulted, only that it had sounded Indian. Was she dark-skinned like me? I wondered if Mr. Samuels saw her when he looked at me.

I tore off my gloves and started to enter the orders into the computer. I asked the clerk to page Surgery so I could give them a heads-up. As I waited for the call back, I stared into my coffee, remembering how slowly I had stirred in the half-and-half as Mr. Samuels's legs had twisted in pain, how painstakingly I had added the sugar, almost grain by grain, as his intestines pushed against his testicles and his scrotum ballooned. To the patient, those six minutes of procrastination on my part must have felt like an eternity. While he certainly deserved to pay for his past violent behavior, it wasn't for me to decide when or how. In my mind, this wasn't the time.

The surgeon, Dr. Castellano, was just leaving a patient's

room on the floor. She said she would swing by to take a look, as the shift might change by the time Mr. Samuels's test results came back. Five minutes later, she was in and out of the patient's room.

"Yeah, Dr. Harper, pretty impressive. Please give a call once the labs and CT are done. If I haven't heard from you before my shift is over, I'll let Dr. Ritter—she's the day doc— know to expect your call."

Fate had delivered this man into the care of three female doctors that evening, each of whom had calmly gazed at his excruciatingly swollen genitals. Women were the ones to inspect him, to touch him, and, ultimately, to slice open his flesh to save his life. Was any of this irony lost on him? From that experience, did he learn how it felt to be vulnerable? I wondered if it might expand his definition of gender, what it meant to be female or male. I wanted to believe that he would never grab a woman again, and I took another moment to stand there trying to convince myself that this could be true. Probably not, but maybe.

I'd update the surgeons with the details of his CT, which would confirm his strangulated hernia, so they could better plan his case for the OR to remove the dead bowel and close up the deficit in his fascia that had allowed the breach so that now his body was busted like his character.

If Mr. Samuels were ever to evolve, it would be due to experiences like this one, where people who didn't have to care for him chose to do so anyway, regardless of his past actions. And, yes, people who commit the type of violence that Mr. Samuels did should be held accountable by the appropriate people, in the appropriate ways. Still, his life lessons were for him alone to choose to learn from or disregard as he decided.

If I were to evolve, I would have to regard his brokenness genuinely and my own tenderly, and then make the next best decision. My choosing to care about his welfare, my decision to hold in my heart the best intention for another human being no matter who that person is or what they have done, that day in the ER, despite my disgust at his previous behavior and the possible moral decay that had led him to it, was a social action.

Two more patients flashed on the board, a sore throat and eye discharge, but they would wait just a little while longer while I finished with Mr. Samuels.

FIVE

Dominic: Body of Evidence

"JUST MAKE HIM DO IT!" A voice rang out, followed by the sound of metal grating on metal.

I leaned past my computer screen toward the triage area to see a young man in handcuffs chafing at the bony prominences of his reddened wrists. Fading charcoal gray lines of graphic tattoos on his left forearm were almost indecipherable against his dark skin.

"I didn't do nothing!" the prisoner shouted.

"That's enough out of you!" a police officer commanded.

"Listen, we have to take your vital signs. Put on this gown." The voice was from Carl, the charge nurse assigned to head the nursing team for the shift.

"I ain't doin' nuthin'. I don't want to be here. I don't want to put on that gown. I'm not doin' nuthin'." The young man looked away—away from the charge nurse who tried to stare at him straight in the face, away from the officer who looked only at the nurse, away from the audience comprising the full ER occupants, who were intently watching the show.

His white shirt, made brighter still by the contrast of his chocolate skin, quivered with every shallow exhale. His dark jeans were clean and fit perfectly, as if he had just been wearing them on a Diesel runway. His white trainers weren't new, but they were certainly well cared for—bright, clean, polished. He couldn't have been more than five foot nine and looked thin and frail under his fashionable attire.

The four officers who brought him in seemed like overkill—like rolling in military tanks to secure a small-town demonstration. At the same time, I can't claim with absolute certainty that the show of force wasn't indicated: I've seen a 125-pound man on PCP evince Herculean strength that required everyone in the emergency department to subdue him with injectable tranquilizers and physical restraints. I always felt bad watching a patient being wrestled to the floor, knowing that he could be injured, knowing that, heaven forbid, he could be killed, even though we were doing it for his protection and ours. Even when everyone has the best of intentions, things can go terribly wrong. Yes, the patient had chosen to take the PCP, necessitating that the authorities be called and he be brought to the ER, thereby involving us in the danger of his personal decisions. Although, in so many ways, we in the ER pay the price for a patient's choices, it never feels okay when there is a complication. Because the stakes are so high, the moment we decide we have to go hands-on, the critical action is always contained in the question before: Is this truly necessary?

"You're gonna have to make him do it," one police officer said to Carl. "He has to be examined, so you're just gonna have to make him comply."

I shifted my chair to keep one ear and one eye on the commotion, eavesdropping as I clicked away at my computer. This section of the ER was circular, with the doctor's station in the middle, so it was possible to keep an eye on most rooms. The situation didn't appear to be defusing, so I knew I needed to wrap up my work and head to triage.

"What's his name?" Carl asked.

"Dominic," the same officer replied.

"Dominic, you're gonna have to put on this gown and let us examine you," Carl said firmly.

"I ain't doin' nuthin'. These cops are lying. I didn't do nuthin' and I don't want to be examined. I don't want to be here," he exclaimed as drops of spittle flew from his mouth.

As if suddenly resigned, his face became a mask of calm, but that flying spittle told another story.

"Someone, please get the doctor," an exasperated charge nurse entreated.

Hearing this, Lauren, the second-year resident who was my charge for that day, took five hurried steps over to the melee. Lauren's steps were always hurried and overconfident. She was pale white, of average height, with a narrow nose and a frame as slender as her fine mousy blond hair, which fell limply in a taut ponytail at the nape of her neck.

She would have been entirely nondescript if not for the salience of her habitual condescension. She, like me, had heard the drama unfold. I was the only attending physician on in my section and just wanted three precious minutes to finish up with the last five cases before delving into this quagmire.

I could practically hear Lauren put her hands on her hips as she asked, "What's going on here? I'm Dr. Morgan. What seems to be the issue, officers? Carl?"

I took a deep breath, knowing that she would not be the one to resolve this situation. I just needed 170 more seconds to wrap up my work so I could smooth things over in triage. I also knew that I had to give Lauren a chance to at least attempt effective mediation. She was, after all, my trainee, and thus my obligation for the next nine hours, forty-seven minutes, and thirty-two seconds.

I took a deep breath for another reason: I wanted so badly, when I entered the triage area, to see black officers and a white prisoner, or at least one black officer and a non-black prisoner—anything other than the stereotypical white cop/black prisoner scenario. But I had already surveyed the scene, so I already knew—I made myself take another breath—that in triage was the configuration of characters I least wanted to see.

We are not yet at a time in America when the attributed or perceived actions of a brown or black or queer or Muslim "wrongdoer" are considered singular. Instead, such accused are seen as emblematic of an entire demographic, one labeled guilty before charged. And yet, the overwhelming majority of spree killers from the most notable mass shootings in U.S. history are male and white. The crimes of each of these assailants are repeatedly viewed as individual acts indicative of one sad, tormented man's mental state and not of his entire gender and certainly not of his race. This privilege of individual self-determination is purposefully not extended to all. Strangely but not coincidentally, these massacres do not lead to large-scale examinations of the state of "maleness" or "whiteness" in America—both topics that Americans most desperately need to examine.

It could not be delayed any longer. I stood up and removed my gray fleece and put on my long white coat. At that time in my career, I always had my white coat with me. In truth, I used it more to hold a collection of medical references and my favorite pen light, which had pupil measurements on its side, than to show everyone that I was a doctor. In fact, I almost never wore it. I found it cumbersome to run around an ER wearing a long coat with full pockets. And indeed, it became a liability in the department: just another item I had to protect from blood, vomit, and bedbugs. But apart from what I could stash in its pockets, there were times when it was a useful costume. Sometimes I had to explain to a family member that her courageous mother had just passed away, or ask another if his father's end-of-life wishes included cardiopulmonary resuscitation. The coat was my garment of choice for such conversations. It was a uniform that signaled expertise, authority, confidence. And now here was another scenario in which I had found it came in handy.

As I approached, Lauren was looking directly at the patient and saying, "Sir, you are going to have to do what we say. You did something that is dangerous and life threatening. Now you are under arrest. You must get in this gown, and then we will examine you." No invitation, no question. Simply her interpretation of the events and a directive to comply.

No one moved.

Suited up, I approached the stalemate. I looked at the patient's face. He was turned away, looking at nothing in the far corner of the room. His chin was tilted upward, his jaw tight, his brow glistening with the first signs of perspiration. His breathing was rapid and shallow.

I clasped my hands in front of my chest. "Hello, sir," I said softly. He lowered his head to look at me. I was anywhere from twelve to four inches shorter than everyone else in the area. He and I were at least ten shades darker than everyone else in the triage room. "Sir, what's your name?"

His jaw loosened just enough for him to say, "Dominic."

"Yes. And your last name?" I asked.

"Thomas. Dominic Thomas."

"Hello, Mr. Thomas. I'm Dr. Harper. I'm the doctor in charge here, so I just have to ask you a couple questions. I'm sure they're the same ones everyone else has asked you.

Please just bear with me. Can I first ask you why you're in the emergency department today?"

"I don't know. I didn't do nuthin'," he said, his voice rising. I saw his neck and shoulders begin to tense and his arms extend behind him. Nearly shouting, he continued, "They arrested me and brought me here for nuthin'."

Officer Quigley, one of the four large white officers standing around the patient, spoke up. "Dominic here is under arrest for drugs. We raided the house and saw him swallow bags of drugs when he was trying to flee the scene. That's why he's here. We need you to examine him and get the bags out."

Turning back to Dominic, I asked, "Mr. Thomas, did you swallow bags of drugs?"

He sucked his teeth and then replied, "No! They don't know what they talkin' 'bout!"

I looked back at the officer who'd spoken. He rolled his eyes and looked away.

"Mr. Thomas, of course I have to make sure you understand that if you or anyone swallowed bags of drugs, it is really dangerous. The bags could cause a blockage in your bowels. Even worse, they could leak and cause all sorts of things like heart attack, an inability to breathe, pain, and even death."

"I got it, miss, but I didn't do it, so it's not an issue."

"Okay, can I just ask you a couple more questions? It'll be fast."

"Yeah."

"Do you have any medical problems?"

"No."

"Do you take any medications?"

"No."

"Are you allergic to anything?"

"No."

"Any surgeries?"

"No."

"Any alcohol or drugs today?"

"No."

"And my last question. Mr. Thomas, would you like us to examine you today?"

"No. I wanna get outta here."

"Okay, then we will discharge you."

At this, the officers bristled. Officer Quigley exclaimed, "We brought him here for an examination. You have to examine him. That's the procedure."

"What procedure are you referring to?" I asked. I didn't accept what the cop was telling me, and I questioned why he felt comfortable instructing me to do anything at all.

"Ma'am, we do this all the time," he said, sighing. The sigh telegraphed to me that this man, this older, taller, heavier white cop, felt I was both missing a critical point and wasting his time.

"Oh, do you all have a court order for us to examine this man against his will?" I asked, implying that this must surely be the missing piece of information.

"No, but he's under arrest for a crime."

"I do understand what you're saying, but it is against the law to force a medical examination on a competent adult human being. If you don't have a court order, I would be breaking the law to do further medical evaluation on this man against his will. So, if Mr. Thomas does not want a medical examination, there will be no medical examination, because this is his right and this is the law in the entire United States of America."

Officer Quigley, the charge nurse, and the resident all stared at me. Then they began to explain to me that other physicians had forced such exams on patients.

"I'm sorry to hear that," I told them. "I'm sorry to hear that there are doctors who will break the law for this reason. I am not one of those physicians."

Lauren turned around and went back to her desk.

Carl, whose face communicated total disbelief, asked, "So we're just gonna let him go, with no triage or anything? Because he wouldn't even let me triage him."

I turned back to the patient. "Mr. Thomas, is it okay to just take some quick vital signs on you? Just a couple of things like your blood pressure and heart rate? I promise it won't even take two minutes. As long as your vitals are okay, we'll get you right out of here."

"I'm not putting on that gown." He scowled.

"You don't need to change for this at all."

"Okay, go 'head."

"Thank you."

I turned to Carl. "Excellent. I already got the history, so

triage is done. He refuses any examination, which is his prerogative, so I'll start on his discharge papers now. Just give a yell with those vitals when you get them."

I turned away from the triage area, the dumbfounded police officers, and the annoyed charge nurse. I overheard nurses on both sides of the department debating the ethics of my letting the prisoner go. I heard them telling stories of how it was common hospital practice to make an intervention; of how just the other day Dr. Brisbane, another ER doctor, had placed an NG tube up the nose of a patient, down the back of his throat, and into his stomach to pump gallons of GoLYTELY, the fluid used in a colonoscopy prep, into his gut until his stool ran clear, to remove the alleged drugs from his system. This was the first I'd heard of this frankly horrifying malpractice. Because attending physicians in the ER tend to work in parallel to each other, with their sole focus on expediting the care of their individual patients, the only time I got wind of what my colleagues were up to was during sign-out or through rumor.

This work just got harder. While practicing medicine was feeling increasingly crucial personally, between the hospital bureaucracy and the colleagues who brought their limited perspectives to work—they were, after all, only human—the prospect of it being a sustainable career path for me was diminishing.

As I listened to the war stories of heroic medical efforts on unwilling captives, Maria, a feisty Latina transplant from the Bronx, chimed in. "Yeah, well, Dr. Harper is correct.

You cannot force an examination on anyone just because the police or family member or any third party happens to request it. We need to treat people like human beings. I'm tired of people treating certain people like animals."

I wanted to stand up and second everything Maria had just said, but I already had, in my management of the case. Besides, I needed a rest from standing, knowing that just seconds after I finished wrapping up Dominic's case, I'd have to stand up again. For those few moments, I typed. To the extent it was possible, I'd stay out of the line of gossip. I leaned toward Lauren, who was positioned at the computer station just in front of mine. "Don't worry about this case. I'll write him up. Just move on to the next patient. Nothing for you to do here, since I already took care of it."

Lauren looked at me with her typical antagonism. "Are you sure? I can write it up. I'm actually waiting for a callback from Hospital Ethics. I told them the whole case because I don't think he can refuse an exam and medical interventions. We really need the Ethics Board in on this one if you're going to let him go. I've worked with Dr. Linden and Dr. Jacobson on similar cases, and we just tell the prisoners what we are going to do. They don't have a choice. I don't understand what you're doing." Her tone was more indictment than question. It was the tone she used to assert that she knew more than I did, and for reasons she would never have dared articulate.

It was the very fact that Lauren felt comfortable assuming greater inherent wisdom on the part of the white, male physicians Linden and Jacobson that might have horrified her to examine in herself. For these same reasons—their white privilege—she would have followed their instruction anywhere, even if they directed her to literally break the law. While she wouldn't have spoken the words, her *tone* communicated one of the ubiquitous microaggressions faced by people of color and the *content* of her words showed how such a microaggression is inextricably linked to the gross aggression that follows.

Although I had been having issues with Lauren over the past sixteen months we had worked together, it occurred to me that, in this moment, she was being entirely honest. Yes, there was her typical peevish passive-aggressive tone, but I saw now that she genuinely didn't understand. I knew her only within the confines of work, so I couldn't pretend to know why she hadn't considered these issues more deeply. Certainly, there was a type of privilege in it. Willingly or not, Lauren had donned the cloak of white male privilege, and it fit snugly over her own skin. After all, this is the only way oppression can function: It requires the buy-in of a certain percentage of those it actively oppresses in order to pit those groups of subjugated people against one another.

I thought about the powerful underlying assumptions that had made it so easy for the police to transport this patient to a hospital and for his sovereignty to be taken away. It could be related to his dealing drugs—though, we see all sorts of patients with drug-related issues, and they are not typically brought to the emergency department in chains.

And there is certainly no expectation that we will simply accept that their bodies should be violated because of their alleged illegal drug use.

But for Dominic, it seemed somehow warranted, somehow a commonplace, that his rights as a patient should be tossed aside. I looked at him; his autonomy was so provisional. But then, had he ever had self-determination? Had he even been considered to have ownership of his black body? There was no medico-legal reason for a doctor or a hospital to usurp his decision-making capacity, and yet, for some people, it was expected. In the face of these truths, we are reminded that for many people, their bodies are not considered their own. For those whose bodies are viewed as suspect and threatening, those bodies, at the preference of a more privileged body, could be manipulated, even assaulted.

As I stood there in my white coat, I was reminded of Dr. J. Marion Sims, often referred to as the father of gynecology, who in the nineteenth century conducted experimental surgeries on enslaved women. The women, who had hopes of treatment from a purportedly competent physician, instead were pinned down on operating tables screaming in agony while he sliced into their pelvic regions without the benefit of anesthesia. Sims continued to torture enslaved women in these barbaric ways until he felt he'd perfected his techniques and felt comfortable performing them on white women, but in their case, with the humane addition of anesthesia.

I was reminded also of the Tuskegee syphilis experiment, in which for *forty years*, beginning in 1932, the U.S.

Public Health Service recruited 600 black men, 399 of them with syphilis, ostensibly to offer them treatment for "bad blood." The men with syphilis were intentionally denied treatment so that the U.S. government could study the progression of the disease over the course of their lives and then autopsy them after they had died. Not only were the men in the study not informed of their disease or treated for it, but steps were taken to prevent them from receiving treatment elsewhere; for example, STD clinics were provided with a list of study enrollee names so that they would be refused treatment should they have sought it. The long-running study was not put to an end until 1972, when public pressure led to a federal investigation that deemed the Tuskegee syphilis experiment unethical.

I was reminded, too, of Dr. Albert Kligman's experiments on imprisoned men in Philadelphia from the 1950s to the 1970s. Kligman biopsied, burned, and deformed the bodies of prison inmates to study the effects of hundreds of experimental drugs. Men were subjected to such atrocities as inoculation with herpes, gonorrhea, and various carcinogens. Kligman went on to become a millionaire after co-developing the popular acne medication Retin-A via his studies on inmates, while many of his victims were left with chronic medical conditions that irrevocably damaged their organ systems.

While significant advances have been made in areas of racial equality, we still have miles to go. That day in the ER, Dominic was evidence.

"Lauren," I asked, "do you know what 'treating' this patient would entail? We would be commanding him to have an examination he doesn't want. We would have to restrain him in some way—physically and/or chemically. We would then put a needle in him to draw blood. We would force him to have an X-ray. If the X-ray didn't show anything, and it probably wouldn't, then we would force him to have a CT. We would have subjected this man to two studies of radiation to pacify law enforcement, who have no legal right to force anything on his body. Who would be legally responsible if there were an adverse event from these refused medical interventions? Not to mention who would be legally responsible for the physical assault that a forced examination would entail? You don't even know if the police are telling the truth. Why is any of this acceptable? Furthermore, even if he did swallow drugs, he is an adult who is competent and sober, and who is medically and legally allowed to make his own decisions. We can't force parents of children to allow immunizations that prevent epidemics of devastating pediatric disease; we can't force a hemorrhaging Jehovah's Witness to accept a blood transfusion; we can't force someone having a heart attack to go for a life-saving cardiac catheterization if he refuses it. You know all these things. We have all had these very cases and simply signed the patients out against medical advice. Why would this be different, even if there is a potential life threat?"

Lauren stared at me in silence, her posture perfect. She gently chewed her lower lip.

I heard the clerk call out, "Anyone waiting for Hospital Ethics?"

Lauren waved vigorously at the clerk to send the call to her phone.

I watched and waited while she was on the phone. She didn't say much, just a series of "ohs" and "ahs." Then: "I see . . . really? Okay, well, thank you for your help."

I sat still at my computer, attempting to breathe in for a count of three and out for a count of six (or something like it), to dampen the disgust as my anger mounted—anger that my resident, my privileged, highly educated white female resident, had felt comfortable being so disrespectful as to dismiss my judgment on this matter; that she had felt she had the right to invoke what she deemed a higher authority: older white doctors who'd done the police's bidding in the past or whatever voice happened to be on the other end of the line from Hospital Ethics.

I looked down at my hands on the keyboard, my slender, dark brown hands, dry from constant washing and dousing with alcohol-based sanitizer between patients. As I noted the contrast of my dark wrists extending from the cuffs of my stark white coat, I was reminded of which costumes in America, even in the twenty-first century, are seen as legitimate and which are not.

I recalled the conversation with my department chairman that morning. I had sunk uncomfortably into the plush leather couch across from him. Part of me awaited congratulations upon my promotion to a new hospital position. The other part, the part that felt weighty and awkward sitting three inches deep on this sofa, anticipated the speech he would inevitably make. It was the same speech he'd had to make several times before, to the other women and black physicians who left before I had arrived at Andrew Johnson Hospital:

"Michele," he said. "You know every time I try to make a change at this institution, I just can't. I'm always blocked. You didn't get the position. I'm sorry to say it. You're qualified. I just can't ever seem to get a black person or woman promoted here. That's why they always leave! I'm so sorry, Michele. They've decided that even though you were the only applicant, and a super-qualified one at that, they're just going to leave the position open. I'm so sorry. I hope you'll hang in here with me anyway."

His words had hung sadly between us. He had spoken with the heavy heart of a longtime liberal white man who would shake my hand, smile, close the door behind me, and then sit back down in his comfortable, secure chair. His effort was complete. His part was done. I was the one left to live with the limitations of that bigotry. I was the one left to get up and fight for Dominic and myself.

America still has so many more strides to make. I am evidence.

Lauren turned to me. "Well, the hospital ethicist says that she reviewed this case and even spoke to Legal about it. Turns out it's true that we can't force any evaluation on this patient. Well, good to know. I'm gonna go see this little kid with a cold." She closed her computer screen and headed over to Room 5.

I typed an extremely brief note on Mr. Thomas and swiveled in my chair to let Carl know the papers for his discharge were ready. Then I waved good-bye to Mr. Thomas; he gave me a barely perceptible nod and then continued to stare into space. Officer Quigley grabbed the discharge papers from Carl and mumbled something about everything being so ridiculous. The officer swept his arm across the room in the direction of Mr. Thomas. "Go 'head," he said, in a manner that decisively conveyed his utter contempt for what had just unfolded.

What we had just experienced had offered an opportunity for all of us to recognize that America bears not just scars, but many layers of racial wounds, both chronic and acute. In order to move beyond them, we need to look at them for what they are, diagnose them, treat them, heal them, and then take care not to pick at the scabs, reopening the old wounds and creating new ones. I know how hard it is to stand and look at tortured and infected flesh. I know because it's part of my job, and therefore something I cannot choose to look away from: soft skin splitting, macerated by brutality and time, half-eaten by maggots spilling out the sides, noxious gases spurting from the extremity of our trespasses. We need to stand face-to-face with it, to look and feel and smell and taste what we do, so we can choose exactly how we want to be in this world.

Just as we needed to look at the body of Emmett Till, the

fourteen-year-old black boy who was murdered in 1955 by two white men who had accused him of flirting with a white woman while visiting relatives in Mississippi. They kidnapped the child, beat him, gouged out his eyes, shot him in the head, tied a cotton gin fan around his neck with barbed wire, and then threw his mutilated body into the Tallahatchie River. His mother insisted on an open casket at his funeral, so all of America could see how the nation treated its children, how we treated each other, how we were in this world.

Dominic Thomas brought me back to the reason I had chosen to become a physician: Being a healer is the powerful gift of bearing witness in an authentic way that allows us to mindfully choose who we are. In this way, there is another path.

I choose to witness the tortured flesh. I support it in my hands and cleanse the wounds as gently as I can. I apply intention and salve to heal. I write about these moments so we always remember the power of our actions, so we always remember that beneath the most superficial layer of our skin, we are all the same. In that sameness is our common entitlement to respect, our human entitlement to love.

I hit Send on the email I was writing, packed up my stainless-steel water bottle, coffee mug, and uneaten granola bar, and tucked them all back into my lunch bag. I wanted to leave the day behind me.

Once home, I shed my scrubs and then showered, rinsing off the shift. Dressed in a robe, I propped my feet up on the ottoman, and my shoulders floated down to settle into the sofa. My boss had probably received and responded to my resignation letter by now. There was comfort in knowing that this was the end of the road here. My chair would give me the time I needed to line up another job before I left.

And so, I started the process of beginning again. I knew that there must be another place where, as a doctor, I could both practice medicine and climb the administrative ladder. After all, I was here to ascend. I was here to help as many people as I could . . . somehow.

SIX

Jeremiah: Cradle and All

MONTEFIORE HOSPITAL in North Philadelphia was my next stop. Here there was career mobility. Montefiore was like Mercy Lite. In this way, it was a homecoming of sorts, and like any homecoming, it was a temporary return to the nest to celebrate what was, to visit the comfortable haunts— old lovers and friends who used to fit before I molted into this new skin.

There were several similarities to my residency experi- ence at Mercy Hospital in the South Bronx. Montefiore had a volume of more than 95,000 patients a year, and Mercy had more than 145,000. At Mercy, I had been a chief resident. In the Montefiore health care system, I was one of the assistant medical directors. Because I was hired to move into the di- rector position at one of the hospital's suburban locations, I was setting meeting agendas, writing protocols for treating high-risk medical conditions (such as acute stroke and heart attack), assisting in provider evaluations for staff, and sending out my own emails on blood cultures and medication documentation.

Prior to starting the position, I hadn't fully realized that sending such emails in the role of assistant medical director didn't make the work feel any more relevant. As I sat at my desk in my new position, with a list of administrative tasks about standard operating procedures, proper documentation in medical records, and risk reduction, I remembered the passion that had brought me to emergency medicine in the first place: sitting with people in crisis and helping them take the first steps toward healing. Mercy Hospital had stoked the fires of this passion and had prepared me well to address the challenges faced by the Montefiore population.

Our mission at Mercy had been to serve the community in a competent and culturally sensitive way, regardless of patients' ability to pay. It was an especially noble mission, given that the population in the South Bronx was as hardworking as it was poor; in fact, at that time, it was home to the poorest congressional district in the nation. One-third of the patients the hospital treated were entirely uninsured, and many residents didn't have a primary care physician. So, when the free clinics in the neighborhood were too busy or closed, we were literally their only hope for care.

Suffering from everything from gunshot wounds to malnutrition to stroke, patients lined up for triage at Mercy. Violence in this neighborhood was as regular as leaves falling in October, and its roots lay in battles over money, respect, self-esteem—all fed by deep notions of not having enough, not feeling enough; by geysers of frustration and hurt.

I remembered the moment during residency when I first realized the brambly nature of this violence and these social webs. At that time, the ER at Mercy was divided into sections: Adult Medical, Adult Surgical, Follow-up (for wound checks, suture removals, etc.), and Pediatric. On that particular day during my second year of training, I was working in the pediatric side of the emergency department. The next chart on the rack read, "13 yo male, head trauma."

I scanned the triage notes: normal vitals, no medical history, a blow to the head. I tapped on the open door and introduced myself to the child, named Gabriel, and the two adults who appeared to be his parents. The boy sat at the side of the stretcher with his hands folded in his lap, his eyes fixed on his interlaced fingers. Behind him, a cartoon of a herd of purple elephants with rising red balloons decorated the wall. Mom stood near the cabinet, arms resting over her purse. Her hands were leathery and her mouth soft. Dad sat in the chair next to the stretcher. His eyes were weary, and an earthy odor emanated from his clothes.

I started by collecting the requisite information: past medical history, vaccination history, medications, allergies to medications, and so on. Then I moved to the matter at hand. The child told me that a classmate, "T," routinely harassed him at school, picking on him about his appearance and threatening him. T was larger than Gabriel and part of a rough crowd. Gabriel didn't know if the other boy was in a gang, but T's crew seemed to be in and out of school as much as juvenile detention.

I asked what had happened, and Gabriel relayed the following story. He had earned good grades on his report card, was helping care for his little sister, and had completed all his chores, so his parents rewarded him with the sneakers he'd wanted for his birthday—popular and pricey shoes, which he proudly wore to school the next day. On his way there, T cornered him in the empty lot next to the school grounds and demanded that he hand over the sneakers. Gabriel refused and continued walking. T followed him, and Gabriel started to run. T then jumped on Gabriel, pulled him to ground, and proceeded to punch him about the head and body. Gabriel tried to defend himself, but the other boy pulled a knife and threatened to kill him, adding that Gabriel was lucky he didn't have his gun on him that day. Terrified, Gabriel removed his shoes. T picked up the sneakers, spat on Gabriel, cursed, and walked away. After T left, Gabriel ran home shoeless on the hot, cracked pavement of the South Bronx.

He had not passed out, had not experienced nausea or vomiting, and had no abnormal sensation to his skin or any weakness. No neck pain, no difficulty breathing. He had visible swelling and redness on the left side of his face, his shoulders, and chest, and superficial abrasions and cuts to his feet.

What struck me about Gabriel was how quiet he was as he lay down on the stretcher for his examination. What's remarkable about children is how receptive and resilient their bodies are: They are more likely to bend than to break. Even if a liver tears, oozing hemorrhage from blows to the abdomen, or a blood vessel bursts behind the eye from forceful shaking, nothing is evident on the surface but the beautiful cinnamon skin of their bellies, a regular pulse at their soft wrists, and normal color in their big, bright brown eyes. Kids don't have the language to name the pain, neither physical nor psychic, nor the resources to address it. Just like adults, children house spiritual pain inside, where it sloshes around vital organs. But in children, the effects of trauma are stickier, shaping the contours of their viscera, the depth their diaphragm respires, the way their heart chambers fill.

"Okay, Mom and Dad, I just have to ask Gabriel a couple of questions alone," I said, knowing I needed to complete the imperative abuse screen for any child presenting with injuries. Gabriel's story made sense and sounded credible, but all too often the assailant can turn out to be a family member or another adult the child knows.

After Mom and Dad had left the room, I told Gabriel he could sit up, now that the physical exam was done. Then I pulled a chair up next to him and said, "Gabriel, I am so sorry about what happened. It is terrible and unfair. That shouldn't happen to anyone."

Gabriel nodded once and stared down at his thumbs.

"Gabriel, I have to ask you some questions, to make sure you're safe. Just so you know, everything we speak about is confidential. If it turns out that you're in physical danger, then that's when I'll need to break confidentiality. It's only because we have to make sure you're safe. I want you to know that I won't do anything behind your back. We'll talk, and I'll tell you if we are in an area where we have to involve other people in the discussion. Okay?"

"Okay," he mumbled.

"We ask these questions of all young people, and even all grown-ups, because sometimes people are hurt by people they love, like family members, friends, teachers. Know what I mean?"

"Yeah," Gabriel replied.

"Who do you live with?"

"My parents and little sister."

"How old is your sister?"

"She's seven."

"Do you like your little sister?"

"Yeah, she's cool. I mean, she gets on my nerves some-times, but she's my sister."

"Yeah, she has to do that, right?" I said, chuckling a little and meeting Gabriel's smile. "I hear you take good care of her, don't you?"

He nodded.

"Do you get along with your mom and dad?" I asked.

"Yeah."

"Do you feel safe at home?"

"Yeah."

"Does anyone at home ever hit you? Or threaten you when you get in trouble or something?"

"No. I mean, I be put on punishment if I don't do what I'm supposed to do sometimes, but nothing like being hit or anything."

"And how's school?"

"It's okay."

"Do you have a favorite subject?"

"Not really."

"Do you like going to school?"

"Not really."

"Why not?"

"So many problems there. Always drama. Always fights."

"Do you feel safe at school?"

"Nah, but I'll take care of things."

"What do you mean?"

"I mean I will take care of things. This won't happen again."

"What do you mean?"

"Miss, I mean, I'll handle it."

Almost reflexively, I asked the question I didn't want to ask because I didn't want to know the answer. It was so much easier to choose to believe that the possibility of escalation didn't exist here; easier to believe that this boy would leave the hospital and be able to go to school safely and survive to graduation; easier to believe that he didn't literally feel his life was in danger every time he left his home or that his fear was somehow off base. I could have chosen to believe that and simply have posed a leading question—*Okay, so you mean you're fine? Everyone will be okay, right?*—and he would have had the opportunity to nod in tacit agreement. We could then have been contentedly linked in a comfortable lie—a lie, like any lie, that would have required the active participation of both parties.

But I didn't do that. Instead, I let the question jump from my lips. (I can't claim any great insight in asking it. It felt more as if I were on the edge of my seat while watching a film on HBO and had just blurted out what I most feared right before my friend shushed me, "quiet!")

"Are you planning to get even with him?"

Gabriel replied, "I'm just gonna take care of myself. If he leaves me alone, won't be no issues."

He sat there silently gazing at his hands as he rubbed his thumbs and tapped his foot.

Again, the impulse made me ask him the obvious and seemingly ridiculous next question. It was a question that felt foreign to me, given that I had grown up in Northwest Washington, DC, where people drove Volvos with bumper stickers reading BOOKS NOT BOMBS, COEXIST, and THINK LOCALLY, ACT GLOBALLY. When my classmates parked their BMW convertibles to go to AP English class, they never worried that they would be carjacked. When I walked to my car from my private school, it never occurred to me that I might be threatened for my book bag, loafers, or cashmere sweater.

My lesson on the impermanence of material items was a little different from Gabriel's. Toward the end of high school, I learned that parents can spend more money than they have in order to give the appearance of wealth. But that appearance is belied when one by one bathrooms are rendered unusable because the plumbing can't be maintained and the pool algae is so dense it looks like an extension of the unkempt yard. I didn't know exactly when my family's financial ruin was at its tipping point, but by then, I was well practiced at compartmentalizing.

The job of my youth had been to get out of that house and out of that life. So, when strange men knocked on our doors at all hours, asking for my father (who was invariably not there), and then left, giving no name, no message, I let it go. (Honestly, I was just glad he wasn't home.) And when I heard my mother on the phone mumbling something about legal fees, when my father had to close his medical practice, and when they went on to lose the court battle over house number three in DC, I didn't question any of it. Anyway, my graduation from high school was only months away.

Before my first year of college ended, I knew I could never go back home. Thankfully, my parents' divorce was well under way, and my father was living God knows where. My mother hadn't sued him for alimony—she'd just wanted the marriage over as quickly as possible. But she couldn't afford to maintain that home in any way. Increasingly over that period the house lacked running water and heat. Various animals could be heard scurrying around in the attic. My brother moved out soon after I had, our sister followed, and our mother was at home only sporadically. Fortunately, my grandparents lived nearby. My mother wasn't yet working, so she spent much of her free time at our grandparents' home, but still used our home to sleep, eat, and deal with the final proceedings.

She should have lived with her parents, my grandparents, during this time. Years later, she said her reasoning for not having done so was because she didn't want to impose on them, to crowd their already crowded house, which was also home to my aunt and a cat. But I never found this answer truthful. What's more honest is that for my mother, most topics of discussion—whether it was why she picked abusive men (my brother's father was her first abusive husband; my father, her second), why she valued money over health, where all the money was coming from, and where all of it went—were merely occasions for subterfuge. The real reason she couldn't live with my grandparents was because she couldn't risk their being witnesses to the truth of her life: It had been a sham. Because this truth of her life was a subject she would never broach, rather than risking my grandparents' asking the obvious questions, she stayed in the dilapidated family home. It seemed easier to her, I'm sure, than being exposed to their scrutiny within their four walls. So, my mother preferred to dwell in the dark, in our home, until the matter was forcibly taken out of her hands. This was her well-worn groove.

During my first two years in college, I worked various jobs on campus (at the food court, bartending) to help support myself. My father would send me money, too. I'd siphon off funds from the money orders he sent and from my student jobs to forward to my mother until she had a steady job and had moved out of the District.

During my second year of college, my mother had a yard sale to raise money for herself. I wanted to get back to secure the items I cared about, but she said there wasn't time to wait for a semester break. Besides, she added, someone must have already bought the ceramic fish I made in my favorite high school art class. (I'd fashioned it after one of the fighting fish I remembered from our fish tank, but toned down the hues to black and teal.) And apparently, it was anybody's guess what had happened to the woodblock I carved under the same instructor and the pastoral prints I made from it. Gone, too, were the ceramic mugs I'd made in elementary school.

I was glad when my mother left Washington, but the going was cruel. It felt like the void left after a fire, except there hadn't been a fire. There had just been two adults who'd haphazardly collided just long enough to produce children, create decades of chaos, and then flee, leaving their offspring to pick up the scattered pieces however they could. So, I understood how things got lost and stolen. I "got" the pain of instability. I knew the pain of the kind of violence that happens privately, at home; the violence that's not reported, much less discussed; the violence you can't escape because it's where you lay your head, until you can manage to pack up and secure a safe place to bathe, to eat, to sleep, to be.

Still, *public* violence was new to me. I hadn't grown up with the reality of being unsafe outside the home, of not knowing whether you can walk to the store without being attacked, or go to school without being shot. I had only a hint of this insecurity while growing up with my brother in the 1990s. There were nights when I was worried about his safety driving while black. But that was during an era in DC when black men of affluence were spared the violence wrought upon poor men of color. Those times have since changed; in this one way, our country has moved closer to class equality.

Sure, there were other, rare acts of public violence in my community (a kidnapping in a park, a robbery in a grocery store parking lot), but these incidents were uncommon, so we felt safe at least outside the home if not within.

Still, I read the news and listened to NPR, and theoretically, I knew these things happened. So, a little embarrassed, I asked Gabriel, on that day at Mercy Hospital in the South Bronx, the question I had to ask:

"Do you have a weapon? A gun or a knife?"

"A gun."

I asked again. "You have a gun?"

He said nothing.

I tried again. "Do you have access to a gun?"

"Don't worry about it, miss. Don't worry about it," he replied tersely, indicating that this would be his final answer.

"Gabriel, this is all very dangerous. This is one of those instances I mentioned before, where I have to break confidentiality. Anytime a young person mentions that they have access to a gun and may use it to cause harm, we have to speak with the social worker just to keep you safe."

Gabriel didn't move and didn't say anything. I waited for any response or sign. He simply shook his head and froze.

"I'll be right back," I said.

I went outside and spoke to my supervising attending physician. I presented the case to her—residents must review all patient cases with their supervising attendings—concluding my presentation with my assessment that, given the disclosure of potential violence by firearm, I had to speak with the boy's parents and the social worker. She advised me to proceed. I put a page out to Social Work and then went to the parents, who were waiting outside the examination room. I summarized for them the situation and my concerns.

They looked at me plainly, waiting for the question, waiting for clarification of why I was alarmed.

Now we were all confused. They were stumped by my concern, and I was puzzled by their untroubled stance.

We all went into the room to join Gabriel, who looked up at his parents.

"Miss," his mother said to me, "if he has to defend himself, he has to defend himself."

I paused. The statement was deceptively plain. I was horrified that his parent normalized what sounded like retaliation. It hadn't taken long in my career for me to learn that violence often begets more violence. Each trauma alert, each young person we pronounced, each patient who, if lucky, left the hospital with a colostomy bag, tracheostomy, or wheelchair proved this point. I also knew firsthand that self-defense could make the difference between being memorialized or graduating, and that no child should ever be put in the position to have to make that choice. "Um, okay. This is a very dangerous situation. Anytime we receive information about potential gun violence, we have to get Social Work involved, to ensure everyone is safe," is what came out.

"What are you saying, miss? Are you going to take our son from us?" the mother asked with the first hint of concern I perceived in her voice. The father slumped back in his chair, propped his head against the wall, and sighed, closing his eyes. Gabriel sat up in the stretcher. For the first time during this discussion with his parents, he looked me squarely in the face. His eyes were glassy with disbelief, the way I had looked at the two DC police officers who came to our door and said they would arrest my brother, too, after I had summoned them to stop my *father's* violence. That night, they had communicated to my family that we were all implicated somehow, so all of us would have to pay.

Now, as I stood there looking down at this child, I knew how he felt. I knew that there wasn't anything I could say or do to make him feel otherwise. We were all in this mess together, and none of us would leave feeling vindicated or clean.

"No, that is not the aim here. No one wants to take you away from your family. That will not happen here," I stated, in a desperate attempt to clarify my intentions. As I stood there waiting for the social worker to arrive, I wondered why, in all my growing-up years, no physician had ever spoken to me alone, to ask if I was safe. Neither had a teacher, mentor, or other family member, for that matter. I wondered what might have transpired if they had. I imagine that I, too, would have felt reluctant and scared. I did know that it would have taught me a valuable lesson, one I would have carried with me for the rest of my life: There are adults who will protect another human being. This was something I had to learn later, on my own, once I finally left that house.

The ER social worker, Aisha, arrived and took her report. Aisha was as conscientious as she was fabulously accessorized. While she was undoubtedly a phenomenal social worker, she could have been a notable fashion blogger, too. Each day, she sported her pixie cut with a different selection of dangly earrings depending on her ensemble. How she adroitly walked the hospital halls during her entire shift in four-inch heels as if they were sneakers is still a mystery to me.

When she completed her consultation with the family, she pulled me aside to summarize her findings. She told me that these were hardworking parents who were doing the best they could. Mom worked full time at a grocery store, typically doing overtime to make ends meet. Dad was a janitor, working all hours of the night and day while doing contractor work on the side. They lived in a violent neighborhood riddled with crime. Drugs were sold on every corner, and you tuned out gunshots the way suburbanites tune out the crickets' chorus at dusk.

Aisha placed her hand on my arm. Her tone was kind

but resigned. She didn't break a sweat, and her brow was unfurrowed. Clearly, this was a conversation she had with newbies like me all the time.

"Michele, when you're at war, the rules are different. The members of this family, they're soldiers in a way. They're fighting for their families. The frame of reference in war is different. The atrocities of a war zone are a normal part of life, and you do what you have to do to survive, to make it out, to make it home." She sighed. "You know these are really good people. None of this is right. Gabriel shouldn't think it's okay to use a gun. There are other ways, of course. And he shouldn't feel he has to have a gun to feel safe at school. Schools should be safe. There are other ways for that, too."

She sighed again, this time even more heavily.

"Oh, child," she said, shaking her head. "Anyway, there's no proof that this kid really has access to a gun. No one in his family has one, either. I'll write up my report, and we'll check on the family. There's nothing else to do here." She shook her head again and smiled. "Unless the ER can give these people jobs that are actually living wage and safe places to live." She picked up her clipboard and began to walk away, and then turned to me and asked, "Can we do that, Doc? Lord knows, I wish we could do that. Have a nice day. You know how to reach me!" She waved, turning to see the next patient down the hall.

That was years ago now. I never found out what happened to Gabriel and his family. Yet his story, their story, haunts me.

Now I stood in the trauma bay at Montefiore, waiting to receive the latest trauma notification—all of us robed, gloved, and ready. The call had come in: two young men shot, one in the head, the other in an extremity. When trauma alerts like this one came in, I often thought about how the patient could be Gabriel or so many others like him. It was the beginning of my shift, so I would be taking the more seriously injured one. It's common practice for the fresher doctor to handle any new critical patient. The other doc would head up the less serious injury, in Trauma Room 2, while my team and I were in Trauma 1. We figured the incident was gang-related, but then, that was almost a given.

As I stood at the head of the bed, I checked my suction and laryngoscope blade one last time. One tech was at the foot of the bed with trauma shears, to cut off all clothing for full exposure, so we could check for wounds. Another pulled out a C-collar, a rigid neck brace used to stabilize the cervical spine in any trauma patient where neck injury hasn't been ruled out—just in case EMS didn't have time to place one in the field. One nurse was on either side of the bed, each with an IV setup. The nurse to my right had fluids hanging, the one on my left had monitor leads and the code cart. There were two med students in the room, whispering to each other in eager anticipation. This was their first shift in the emergency room, and they probably already felt like they were in the middle of a popular ER reality show episode.

"Please, just let them get here," I implored. Standing there in the Trauma Room, I could practically feel the charts

building up in the main ER. With a groan, I pinched the top of my mask snug to the bridge of my nose to prevent condensation on my face shield. I stood there thinking about all the things that could go wrong and how I could address them. What if the GSW was to the mouth, and I couldn't intubate? What if it was to the neck, and I couldn't even manage a tracheotomy? There are times, too, when the EMS notification is completely wrong. There was the time a GSW to the chest was called in that was actually a flesh wound to the arm. Who knows? Maybe the guy coming in was only grazed on his scalp.

Nurse Ramirez walked through the Trauma Room doors with an update. "Just a heads-up that y'all will only get the GSW to the head. The other male was diverted to Episcopal, since they're in opposing gangs. The less craziness we have here, the better! They should be here any second."

"Thanks, Chief," Brian, one of the techs, replied.

We heard thunderous rattling at the ambulance entrance. Then EMS appeared, pushing in a gurney with two enormous black sneakers hanging off the edge, kicking in twisting movements. The legs were clad in jeans streaked crimson. Then a torso emerged—a striped shirt with blood dripping down the right side and bits of fleshy matter about the chest. Blood leaking from a pressure dressing to his scalp streaked the floor.

"Sorry, this was a scoop-and-run," one medic announced, beginning his report. "Twenty-something-year-old man. GSW to head. GCS anywhere from thirteen to fifteen. It's

hard to tell because he's agitated. Blood pressure one-ten over seventy, heart rate one-forty, saturating ninety-five percent on room air. We couldn't get IVs. We couldn't tube him in the field."

They parked their gurney next to our stretcher and transferred the patient. One medic began to help Brian cut off the clothes as the other medic continued his stream of information.

"It was just madness at the scene. Sorry for the delay. There was a huge crowd and some fighting still going on. The police had to get us in and out as they secured the scene. Then we just drove like hell to get here."

"What's his name?" I asked as I looked down at the fallen giant on the bed. He had to be at least six foot four and probably 300 pounds.

"Friends said they call him Jay. His ID says Jeremiah; it's with registration." Jeremiah was enormous and thrashing and bleeding from his right scalp.

With swift precision, EMS and Brian cut off his jeans. Bloodstains on the legs, but no injuries. Next, they cut off his shirt. More bloody marks scarring his torso and arms, but no deformity, no injuries, no swelling. There was so much blood. We in emergency medicine do this work every day, but we never entirely numb ourselves to the impact of the body being rent apart to let rivers of life flow from arteries and veins. I couldn't imagine a day when it wouldn't be disturbing to see blood burst forth as if from a broken levee.

I could see no deformity to the neck. Jeremiah was

breathing, he was moaning, he was emitting sounds of anguish. His GCS, or Glasgow Coma Scale, which measures a patient's level of consciousness on a scale of 1 through 15, was somewhere near 15, which was reassuring.

Once he was fully exposed, the nurses placed the patient on the monitor and prepared the IVs. His blood pressure was technically "normal." Given the stress he was under, that was a very bad sign. The constellation of fast heart rate and relative hypotension here signaled that he might have a life-threatening hemorrhage, not to mention the possibility of a catastrophic brain injury. The patient was flailing around, and the EMS guys and Brian grappled to get his legs down. The nurses called the med students over to hold down each arm while they placed one large-bore IV into each antecubital area of his arm, which in lay terms is the crease in the inner arm where the elbow bends. We needed venous access to stabilize him. It was like wrestling with Goliath—an agitated and confused Goliath.

"Jeremiah, Jeremiah, do you hear me?" I called to him softly, placing one palm on his left cheek while inspecting his head. The only wound, which was too much, was the section of his skull that shattered into his brain. Blood oozed from this wound in his right skull around matted chunks of tissue.

"Where am I? Christian! Mom!" he screamed out, thrusting his head from side to side, splattering blood around the head of the bed. His eyes were shut tight as he moaned and cried. A mix of tears and blood streamed down his dark cheeks. His skin was the color of deep mahogany, smooth and rich.

I placed my hands on each side of his head to coax him to stillness. Looking directly down at him, I asked, "Jeremiah, look at me. Can you look at me?"

His eyes cracked open and he looked behind my mask, past my glasses, and into my eyes.

"Can you help me? Please, please help me!" he cried.

"Jeremiah, we are going to help you. Try to be calm. Please try to be still so we can help you," I chanted to him like a lullaby.

"Please, please save me! Moooommmmmm! Please, please save me," he begged as he stared into my eyes.

"Jeremiah, we will help you," I chanted, begging him to believe me, hoping we could both be soothed by my words.

Jeremiah wept. He wept in waves. He wept in howls that stirred the marrow. He wept from a place of pain much deeper than the GSW to his head, pain that hurt more than having bits of his skull shot off and lying on the sidewalk.

"Jeremiah, I am here to help you," I said, gazing between the spaces of his tears as I placed my other hand on his shoulder.

"I'm going to diiiiiiieeeeeeee, I'm going to diiiiiiieeeeee," he gulped in great hiccupping wails.

"We're here for you, Jeremiah." I knew that my words were more important than the medicine I would push into his veins to dampen his consciousness and paralyze his muscles. More important than the breathing tube I would slide down his throat to take control of his breath. More important than the entire surgical team that had been activated for him.

I looked deeper into his eyes and moved my hand to his right cheek to cradle his face because I knew that he was correct. I knew that he was at a crossroads, that he was touching grace. I knew that no matter what he had done to end up in the ER, he deserved to be comforted right now.

"Dr. Harper, we have a line!" reported Trish, one of the nurses.

"Excellent," I said to her, flashing a thumbs-up. "Let's start with lidocaine 150 mg, then 30 mg of etomidate, and 150 mg of succinylcholine," I said, requesting the medications that would relax him so I could perform an endotracheal intubation.

I grabbed my blade and looked into his eyes for the final time. "Now, Jeremiah, you're going to sleep."

After he slipped into unconsciousness I advanced the breathing tube into his trachea and the respiratory team attached the CO_2 detector; we noted good color change, so they placed him on the ventilator. I tore off my bloody gloves to take my stethoscope and listen to his chest: There was good air entry bilaterally, another indicator the endotracheal tube was where it should be. The surgical team flooded the room and whisked Jeremiah off to the operating room. The techs and nurses had moved on to the next patient. EMS loaded up their truck for the next ride. The room was empty save for the aftermath of what had just happened: Monitor leads swung from their screens and plastic needle caps were strewn across the floor along with a mosaic of bloodstains and discarded gloves. I surveyed the scene and was reminded of how these resuscitation rooms are often the most tragic confessionals.

A police investigator came into the room, breaking the silence. He wanted to take my statement: How did the patient present? What was his condition on arrival? What had we done for him in the ER? What was his status when he left the ER?

I answered his questions, we finished the interview, thanked each other for our respective hard work, and stepped over debris to get back to our jobs.

Nurse Esteban met us at the door to say, "Doc, the OR called. That patient coded on the table and died."

The detective heard him. "Okay, now it's a homicide. Thanks, guys," he said as he walked out of the department.

I looked up at Esteban, then I nodded and sighed. It wasn't that I was surprised or confused—it was not surprising that a man who had been shot in the head would die. There was nothing confusing about a man crying out that he was going to die, proving that, in fact, he had perfect insight in that moment. No, my sigh acknowledged the moment he had had with himself and his life, with his blood and his tears, as he was absolved by the bright lights of the trauma bay. It was an understanding that no matter the hand we are dealt at the beginning of our lives, in the end, we face our actions alone. Jeremiah had called out for Mama and for Christian, but in our final moments, everyone we've honored or betrayed is, ultimately, not with us. We lie there alone, flesh and bone, soon to be only spirit.

It occurred to me that maybe Jeremiah was the Gabriel who had picked up a gun. Perhaps it wasn't Gabriel precisely, because maybe he left the ER that day I met him and never touched a gun. Maybe Gabriel left the ER and survived to graduation and was strengthened by the challenges life threw at him. Maybe Gabriel finished college and was now mentoring his teenage sister. Or perhaps he was working toward owning his own business to improve not only his own life, but the lives of those in his family and community.

I suppose it's a matter of faith whether or not we choose our starting ground before we're born into this life. Some begin the journey on flat, grassy meadows and others at the base of a very steep mountain. One path, seemingly smooth, can make it nearly impossible for us to see the ditches and gullies along the way. The other, while painfully tough, can deliver what it promises: If you can navigate that path, you've developed the skills to scale Everest. It isn't fair on many accounts; it simply is. And assuredly, *both* paths include uncertain terrain ahead.

As we place one foot in front of the other, we make choices at every step, no matter the terrain. When we reach the threshold that Jeremiah reached, we look back at our footprints and must face the results of our choices. Alone. In that recognition there is absolution. All deserve the chance to speak and be heard and be touched. If we're lucky, we're touched at every station along the journey, and if nothing else, then at the end.

SEVEN

In the Name of Honor

IF I HURRIED, I could still make the early yoga class. From my condo, it's only a four-block walk to the studio where I cross the threshold from my outer world to the one within. The studio, in the heart of the city, has windows on three sides whereby light stretches through the room. When I arrive, I unroll my mat on the hardwood floor and am bathed in daylight. The flap of the mat's far edge slaps the floor: my personal call to prayer.

Before I take my seat, I press incense powder, called Scent of Samadhi, between my palms and stroke it over my forearms and the tops of my feet. I collect my props (blocks, strap, and blanket), just in case: They sometimes come in handy as an aid to release my tight shoulders or elongate my hamstrings in particularly tricky postures. The scents of sweet and spicy sandalwood and clove root me as I sit cross-legged on the mat. At last I am perfectly still—until the moving meditation begins.

It is on this mat that I learn to let go absolutely, bodily. I let myself be fully present for the fifth sun salutation, and then the sixth, without anticipating whether there will be a seventh. Later, standing in a position named Revolved Triangle, I can see and feel the boundary as my hips fight to splay and my IT band (the thick band of fibers that runs from the pelvis down the side of each leg to the shin bone) screams its revolt. As I slowly and gently support my hips in alignment and refuse to engage the IT band in a fight, the pose blossoms. I take tender breaths and chant my legs into extension so that the fires yield to steam that softens, and my body glides into a deep, cleansing, and previously impossible twist. Revolved Triangle releases into Lunge pose, then I turn my back foot out and down and press the pinky edge of my foot and elongate out through my upper arm into Extended Side Angle. I'm careful to not let the gluteal muscles of my forward leg check out of the game, and knit and then rotate my rib cage up to liberate my trunk and shine my heart upward toward sky.

Then the choice to bind. Does it enhance the pose to twist deeper and farther? Does it enrich the posture to activate the core and draw inward to clasp hands around the body, thereby completing the bind, in Bound Side Angle pose? Can you expand within and beyond this bind while twisting and holding opposite limbs? And most important, can you remember to breathe all the while? These are the questions. This is the choice. The goal is always to breathe deep, sustaining breaths and to decipher which holds at which times will make the experience most nourishing.

Heart leading, I twist back my upper ribs and arm and extend my lower arm under my forward thigh—so difficult for me to maintain side body long as I maneuver my forward arm into position, but I try each and every time. I hold my hands behind me and pull: shoulders back, chest up and back. Extend backward and down through my back hip and foot, extend up and back through my chest and shoulders. Holding strong and long and letting go everywhere else: The wisdom to discern between the two is critical. Never forget to breathe. Always stay present to the gift of breath.

Some days the practice comes easily. Other days, my quads, already weary from yesterday's run, quake from over-exertion. That's when my breath gets caught in my flank and squeezed in my chest. But force is never the way.

Here is where I learn to accept what is in the moment now in order to proceed reverently. Skip the pose and rest if the body needs that moment to replenish, if the breath requires it in order to flow seamlessly throughout the lungs. Pushing hard against contracted muscles will only cause the body to push back or tear. There is a maxim: We're born bound, and we learn to free ourselves. One of my favorite yoga teachers puts it a different way: We are born free, and we choose to bind exquisitely.

It was for this reason that I found yoga soon after I moved to Philadelphia; it was for this reason that I've stayed with it.

There is a saying that every new yogi finds her way to the mat in order to heal an injury. Sometimes the injury is sports-related, though most times it's psychic—perhaps it's a divorce, addiction, or sexual trauma that takes her out of her body as a way to cope when the trauma is too much to bear. After the acute phase of the trauma is survived, it starts to feel safe to integrate the mind and body again. Yoga is a way back to our whole selves. It rejoins the breath, the mind, the heart, and the soul, reuniting the broken pieces into beautiful postures that show us we're rooted in something far greater than pain. The resultant "yoga butt" from regular practice is just a bonus.

On the heels of the New Year and the upcoming stepping down of the suburban site director, whose place I was expected to take, I realized that if I continued this administrative climb, this transition from my role as assistant medical director to that of medical director, I would simply be leaping from one hamster wheel to the next. Sure, I knew I could excel—I was good at my job; I was adept at the treadmill—but as Lily Tomlin says, "The trouble with the rat race is that even if you win, you're still a rat." Now, four years out of residency, after two years at Andrew Johnson Hospital and then another two at Montefiore, I found that this realization had become crystal clear.

My calling is to heal; that is my truth. While medicine's current version of hospital administrative work can be both interesting and valuable, it wouldn't ever bring me closer to being a healer. Most administrative duties involve managing minutiae with the goal of maximizing profits for hospital systems. Second to that is minimizing financial losses. Somewhere far distant to both those priorities is patient care. And way beyond what the mind's eye can see is consideration for the wellness of the providers who are supposed to deliver that care with excellence. I just couldn't be a representative for a mission that was so divergent from my own— even if that meant walking away from the comforts of a higher salary and a better schedule.

I didn't know how I would do it, but I knew I had to rededicate myself to my true path. I knew it meant committing the apparent résumé sabotage of quitting my job, but I also knew that a lack of dedication never yields success. Every part of my being craved alignment. My work, as with everything I do, is a reflection of myself. I practiced yoga to stay on the path. I ate healthily to support my physical body on this journey. I would start meditation to keep my spirit clear. I made it a point to mentor medical students and residents who were women and/or from underrepresented groups of color to make up for the woeful dearth of physician role models for these groups. Medicine still suffers from the same discrimination seen in other fields—women are typically not promoted, while underrepresented people of color are blocked from admittance in the first place. I knew that my emergency medicine clinical work had to focus on underserved populations, as this had always been the medicine closest to my heart. I also knew that my healing work needed to transcend traditional medicine and extend beyond the ER.

For me, the best path was to leave administration. For the

time being, it was also best for me to stop working in academic centers for emergency medicine, which required similar bureaucratic demands and diverted me from my focus on being a healer.

I left Montefiore to dock at the Veterans Affairs Hospital in Philadelphia. Just as I had encountered in my patients at Mercy and Montefiore, I met many heroes while at the VA. Victoria Honor was one of them.

She was steady in her chair, sitting cross-legged, each arm placed deliberately on an armrest, her fingers making soft imprints at the curved vinyl edges. Her grip was tight, her smile at ease. Her hair was parted down the middle, with one goddess braid on each side culminating in a thick rope of loosely kinked hair encircling her head. Springy rings of baby hair peeked out at the edges of her hairline. Her bright, almond-shaped eyes were free of makeup. Actually, she wore no makeup at all, save for lip balm that tinged the air with a hint of citrus. She looked about the same age as I was, both of us appearing younger than our years, but melanin has this effect. Her skin was a shade of moist clay muted by the ill-fitting midnight-blue paper scrubs that hung awkwardly around her shoulders and knees—they appeared to be at least two sizes too big, but they were the smallest we had for the psychiatric patients. This uniform wasn't made for her.

She looked up when I rapped on the door. Leaning

against the wall across from her, I asked why she had brought herself to the hospital.

"Hello, ma'am. I'm here to get cleared. I'm here because it's time for me to get myself together. That's all. It's time." Her smile cracked open, revealing so much hope.

It was strange meeting her here—that's what I remember most. It felt as if I knew her already, as if we could have met as participants in the same noon yoga class on Tuesdays and Thursdays, or as volunteers with the annual Run for Peace 5K. This version of reality—our encounter behind the locked doors of the psychiatric unit in the emergency department— didn't feel right.

"Ms. Victoria Honor . . . by the way, that's a fantastic name!"

She laughed. "Yeah, well, I can't say it was my idea. All thanks to my family. You can call me Vicki."

"Well, Vicki, you sound strong and resolute. Excellent. Yes, I'm here to medically clear you."

This was the standard process for a "psychiatric" patient, whether she was being admitted to an inpatient psychiatric unit for psychosis or being discharged home with a referral to outpatient services for prescription drug abuse treatment. Emergency medicine physicians have to conduct an examination to address any acute medical issue the patient might have before the patient is transitioned to the care of ER psychiatrists or nonmedical specialists.

"And today," I continued, "what are we clearing you from? For?"

She recrossed her legs and raised the index and ring

finger of each hand to her temples. She seemed to be focusing on something far away and hard to see, as if staring at shadows just beyond a noonday sun.

"I have to get my head straight. I went through terrible things in the military. Now it's time for me to get past it all. So, I'm just here passing through to be placed in transitional housing for a while."

"I see." I didn't really, but I said it partially out of habit—the habit of coming into the psychiatric ER and trying to get out as quickly as possible.

Upon badge entry to the locked unit, directly in front and to the right, the first thing you see is an arc of patient rooms. Unlike in the main ER, each room has a hospital recliner chair and most have a flat bed positioned against a side wall as well. Invariably, having opted to keep the lights off, each patient sits there in a separate dark room behind a closed curtain. The tracking board at the nurses' station directly to the right of the unit's entrance lists the reason for each patient's visit, which is almost always some combination of suicidal ideation, homicidal ideation, psychosis, drug dependence, and alcohol abuse. Then you hear the click of the door's metal hardware locking shut, reminding you that the unit is secured. Even after I'd entered this unit hundreds of times, that *click* still triggered in me the instinct to hurry my return to a place where the exit door wasn't locked and the lights were always on.

"I see," I said again. "I'm sorry, but I have to ask you the list of standard medical questions. Some may sound silly, but I just have to ask them for clearance."

She nodded. "Sure, sure. Go 'head, Doctor. I'm here to be honest. I'm here for help, so ask me anything."

"Any recent illness, infection, or anything?"

"No, no. I've been healthy," she replied, knocking on the wood of the bedside table.

"Do you take any medications?"

"Nope."

"Any allergies to medications?"

She shook her head.

"Any recent surgeries?"

I could see Vicki's shoulders melt a little under the weight of her paper scrubs. After a pause, she continued: "No. No recent surgeries." She rocked a little in her seat, moving rhythmically forward and back, touched her breast bone, and then cleared her throat. Then she appended: "Only one, but that was a couple of years ago." She paused and looked at her hand as it lay on her chest, as if it could steady her, as if to remind herself that each word, each disclosure, was part of her process. She looked up and said, "Yes, one surgery, an abortion, years ago now."

"Okay," I responded. It's tough to know when to ask a follow-up question. Clearly, something didn't feel okay. We started off that way, with so much not feeling right about her presence here; her energy told me it had to do with the hesitation she had just displayed.

I told myself that she shouldn't have been sitting there in blue paper scrubs, I shouldn't have been in the psychiatric ER ten minutes before my shift was to end, and the hospital shouldn't have been so packed that ten patients were boarding in the ER (that is, being admitted to the hospital but still waiting for beds to become available on the regular floors). The night doctor shouldn't have been by himself, with me as his only support, and with only a few minutes before the end of my shift, so that he alone would have to care for twenty patients in the emergency department and another ten in the waiting room, because in this hospital, in contradiction to standard practice, it was the responsibility of the ER doctor to care for any boarding patient instead of the admitting in-patient team—the very reason I had ended up feeling guilty enough to see another patient right before I was to sign out and go home. I was here to do medical clearance. Follow-up questions could lead me into a fifteen-minute conversation, and honestly, that was the job of the social worker and psychiatrist. This young woman was the medical picture of health, and that made my job easy.

I continued with the standard questions. "Do you feel you want to hurt yourself or anyone else?"

"Oh goodness, no! No, none of that." She smiled, raised her hand to her neck, and cleared her throat again.

"Now, if you don't mind, just a quick physical exam. May I listen to your lungs and heart?" She agreed, and I completed the perfunctory exam.

"Well, everything's good on my end. All clear! The psychiatrist and social worker should be speaking with you soon. Any questions for me before I go?"

I tucked my stethoscope back on my belt clip and swept

back the rebellious locks of hair that had fallen forward on my face. Vicki watched me lift my deep brown hands to do this. I saw her scan my long, natural hair. I saw her watch me as I tied my dreadlocks to secure them neatly. She got it, and she smiled in gratitude for our similarities.

"No. I'm good." She placed her hands in her lap. "It's nice to see more of us here. I've been here at the VA a few times, and I haven't seen many doctors of color. Before I started going to the new women's health center, I didn't see any women doctors, either. It's really nice to see you. Thank you."

That's why I was there. The VA hospital had a reputation as the place where old doctors went to die. As medicine has evolved over time—or, more accurately, as the business of medicine has devolved over time—many physicians have thought of the VA as their medical home. True, some of the providers at the VA aren't competent enough to practice elsewhere, but that's not the case for all of us. The rest of us come here not out of necessity, but out of choice, to care for those who gave everything with the intention of service to our country and received so little in return. We come here to encounter again that lost heart of medicine. We come here, too, knowing the entrenched legacy of corruption of the VA hospital and still hoping to be at least a small agent of change anyway. While I knew this job would not be my last iteration of healing work, I knew it was an integral part of my path.

The dance of medicine these days is hard. I'm still of the generation that entered medicine to help people, not to be tethered to endless paperwork, bludgeoned by satisfaction surveys linked to nothing except ways to cut pay and staffing, demoralized by the expectation that we see more patients faster—not safer or better, but faster—and then taken to task when patients feel we don't take the time to listen. So, the big consideration in comparing hospital jobs is which set of bureaucratic nightmares will cause the fewest number of sleepless nights. As a hospital-based health care provider, you have the luxury of staying in one job as long as it makes sense—until your provider group loses the contract or you lose your patience. I knew intuitively that the next best choice would come because my growth was ongoing. For the time being, though, I felt deeply that the VA would mark a critical transition point for me.

"Thank you. It is an honor and a pleasure to be here. You're right; we certainly need more. I think with time, little by little, we'll see more positive changes, right? Like most things in history. Just like we're both here today."

We exchanged friendly good-byes, and I pivoted to open the curtain to leave. As I did, I caught a glimpse of her: She had leaned forward in her chair, one hand to her brow, the other tracing circles around a cup of ice water on the table next to her. I looked at her and considered asking The Question. She was entranced by the ice, drawing her fingers across a puddle of condensation on the table, so she didn't notice my hesitation. It was late, so I reconsidered; I just wanted to go home. But I couldn't; I had to ask. I knew the deep well of my sister's pain. Human beings can always know each other if we're still and courageous enough to do so. I, too, had spun in circles and circles of suffering. I had tied myself up in knots in search of liberation. To simply gloss over the violation I sensed in her today made me feel complicit in that silence.

I reclosed the curtain behind me. She looked up, lifted her head from her hand, and smiled.

"Vicki, can I ask you something?" I asked.

"Sure."

"You mentioned you were traumatized in the military. May I ask what happened to you?"

She sat up in her chair and placed both feet on the ground. Putting her hands on her thighs, she rubbed her palms against the crinkled scrubs. When she spoke, her voice was considerably lower than it had been before.

"Yes. Yes, you can." She paused and then resumed the rhythmic rubbing as she looked down at her hands. She made herself stop and then looked up at me. "Remember that surgery I mentioned? The abortion? I was raped in the military."

She didn't cry. Her eyes frosted over—a protective cool. It was the same kind of chill that keeps a person alive far longer than seems possible when she falls into a frozen lake. The kind of cold that slows down the body's metabolic requirements so that the person can live, submerged for hours, in case of eventual survival or, at least, rescue. This is the innate protective wisdom of the spirit: to save the body when it's not yet time to go.

I clasped both my hands to my heart and only partially

contained a full-lung gasp. I didn't have time to realize what I had done. I felt the soul of me unrestrained by the confines of the hospital edifice, Michele, standing next to the me with the VA badge hanging from my neck, Dr. Harper, and half-heartedly tried to pull her back in. "Oh, Vicki. I am so sorry. That should not happen to anyone, anywhere."

This was exactly why I had asked. On some level I already knew, or sensed, what had happened. I also knew that the other part of the atrocity was the silencing. Some would say that the even greater part of the crime was forcing the survivor to hold that trauma alone, knowing that revelation would risk exposing her to blame, judgment, and additional consequences. It was as unfair as it was invalid to blame a victim for the criminal acts of an assailant. The girl I used to be had learned that lesson well in our little glass house in Washington, DC. Only in leaving that house did I come to know in my bones that the peril in being silenced was far greater than that of living loud enough to shatter those walls and bring the whole house down. There is tremendous release in speaking, in letting go of the judgments of others, in the heroism of being willing to heal. It is only in speaking of abuses that we can address them. It is only in speaking of violence that the cycle can be broken instead of replicated day after day in our subconscious, year after year in our lives.

"Yeah. Thank you, yeah." She nodded, releasing deep, depleted breaths.

"It's so good you are healing from this. You're taking control of your life and healing."

"Yeah, I am. It's just one day at a time. You remember when you asked me if I wanted to hurt anyone or myself?"

I leaned against the wall, propping myself up with my hands at my lower back, and readied myself for more. But I didn't know if I could take more right now. I didn't know if I could bear the pain of what she had survived. I didn't know if I could continue to repress my anger in that moment. I didn't know if I could prevent myself from telling her what I really wanted to say: *What they did to you was awful. What they did to you shouldn't be done to any human or any beast. Let's leave this place. I'll introduce you to a social worker and acupuncturist who can help you stay well. And I'll find you a job that will support you. Let's make sure you're out of the military forever. The man who did this couldn't have acted alone. He committed his atrocities because the military allows these crimes within their culture of institutionalized misogyny and toxic masculinity, because our criminal justice system is based on the same, because our nation was founded on these principles first. All of them need to pay the price of full accountability. Come, let's you and me take steps together into change.*

Instead, I steadied my feet and remembered that I was in the psychiatric section of the emergency department of a hospital. This was not my living room; in many ways it wasn't even my life. I had allowed this door to open. In fact, I had opened it, because I was committed to acknowledging Vicki, her experience, and her humanity. I had committed myself to being her provider in this way, so I braced myself for a walk across what was certainly exceedingly hard terrain.

"Yes, I remember," I said.

"Well, I don't want to hurt myself now, but for a long time I didn't want to live. I was all alone over there in Afghanistan. I was the only woman in my unit. I was in Engineering." She paused and brightened. There, for a moment, I caught a glimpse of the Vicki she had probably been before this story. "I could fix anything! I helped to fix the power supplies, maintain the vehicles. I really kept our unit running." Then, suddenly, she was the woman in blue paper scrubs again, sitting there quietly. "I never figured out why, but my sergeant hated me from the very beginning. He would tell me I was nothing, I was worthless." She paused and drew a deep breath into the tiny, hollow shell of herself before whispering, "*Every single day.*"

As she told her story, I began to feel sick. I had that taste that builds at the back of your throat, like stale coffee and two-week-old corn chips, right before waves of acid churn in your stomach to expel a cascade of vomit.

Her eyes met mine and narrowed. "You know, I joined the military because I wanted to do something good for our country and make myself better, too. Then this." She put her hands on her hips and assumed an angry glare. "Private Honor," she barked, impersonating the sergeant, "YOU AIN'T NEVAH GONNA AMOUNT TO NUTHIN'!" She chuckled nervously. "Of course, that's not exactly how he looked, because spit would fly from his mouth when he yelled." Her eyes reddened, and her whole face became heavy. "Can you imagine, Dr. Harper, being told you're worthless every single day by your boss, when you're far away from home? Oh, Doctor, he was just so mean. And he was only mean to me. He would make me stay up at all hours with new tasks for me to do while everyone else slept. You know that when my grandmother died, he didn't let me go home for her funeral. He was supposed to let me go, but he never did. He never let me go." She crossed her arms in front of her and caressed her forearms, rocking herself in the same metrical way as before.

"I am so sorry, Vicki. I am so sorry." My sorrow was filled with a rage that was yielding to a broken heart. I felt sorry knowing that everyone in her story needed healing, but the only person I knew for a fact who had sought it out was sitting in front of me.

She continued: "My grandmother raised me. I never met my father. My mother was around sometimes. She's still alive and has been hooked on drugs my whole life. Well, I guess not the whole time. She just got clean a couple years ago. When she actually does show up, she just asks me for things. Ever since I can remember, it's been the same. When I was ten, she'd ask for the money my grandmother gave me to get snacks at the corner store. She would go into my piggy bank when she thought I was sleeping. I saw her every single time . . ." Her voice trailed off. "My grandmother was the only person I had in the world. She's the one who encouraged me to make something of myself and get an education. But I didn't have the money for college, so I figured I'd join the military first. I'd live with Grandma after that and help her out while I was in school. That was my plan."

The frost in her eyes turned to heat. "You asked me if I wanted to hurt anyone or myself. After my sergeant said I couldn't go to my grandmother's funeral, I wanted to die. I mean, I'm a Christian. I know that suicide is a sin, and I wouldn't ever do it, but I just wanted to die." She shook her head and looked down before continuing. "And then everything just got worse. The sergeant raped me over there in Afghanistan. I was so alone there. I was dealing with that and so alone. Doctor, I couldn't communicate with any of the locals, and there weren't even many locals around where we were, anyway. I never saw anyone. Then another private became my friend. He would bring his food and eat with me when no one else would. I was so thankful when this other private befriended me. Then one night, *he* raped me, too. He stopped talking to me after the attack. Then he had some kind of family emergency—not a death or anything, but a cousin of his was sick or something. They let him go home. He raped me, then they let him go home."

I watched her, a small woman now huddled in a large vinyl chair. All the energy seemed to have drained from her, and for the first time she looked unsteady. She suddenly seemed so far away, far away in Afghanistan, working on artillery, praying for an end to a war that would follow her home.

She slumped back in the chair and expelled two rapid,

shallow breaths. Her gaze was intent while her voice quivered. "Doctor, the other day, the pastor gave a whole sermon on forgiveness. It all sounded like lies. If he had been through what I had . . . If they had had to go through an abortion alone, a pregnancy that came from torture so that I had to get surgery so that my rapist didn't grow inside of me." She continued with her voice rising, "So that they didn't keep taking my body from me, my choices from me. They put me in that position. They took that from me!" Vicki stopped herself. She crossed her arms, then placed her right hand over her mouth. She looked away from me to the lower left-hand corner of the room. She seemed uncomfortable with the anger as if she were concerned with what it might do, where it might go. We both waited there in the space of the pause. I waited for her to make company with a righteous rage. She waited to feel safe. She continued in a tone that was restrained, "If that pastor had been threatened, beaten, and raped over and over . . . I know that Christ wants us to forgive, but I can't. I honestly don't know that I ever can. I want them to die. It hurts me so bad that I just want them to die."

"Vicki, I am so sorry. Your anger makes sense. What they did is horrific." I paused again to give her room. She bit her lower lip and just sat there. "You know you deserve to be happy, right? You know you deserve to be free?"

"Part of me knows. That's why I'm here. I'm here to take my life back. When I first returned from Afghanistan, I started to drink. It was the only way I could be home alone with the thoughts of how it was over there. I couldn't find a job. Even if I could find one, I couldn't get out of bed most days, so what good would that be? It's crazy when you think about it."

"And you don't drink anymore?"

"No, no, I don't. I just got to a point that was lower than when I left for war, lower than anything I could have imagined. I thought of my grandmother. I went to church. One day, I just stopped drinking cold turkey and told myself I had to get better."

"Have you found anyone to be supportive since coming home?"

"You know, my new squad is better. They're the reason I'm here."

"Were you able to tell anyone in your new squad what they did to you?"

"I told my new sergeant and some privates. They all stand by me. Now I have some time off to get better."

"To *continue* to get better," I said, amending her words. "You've already done so much!" I paused, then said, "Did anything happen to the men who raped you? The sergeant who was so abusive?"

"No. They didn't do anything about it; they never do. But my new squad fixed my records. My old sergeant wrote me up for all sorts of crazy things, so I wouldn't get promoted and wouldn't get my benefits, but they wiped all that clean. I have a new therapist, too."

"I'm happy to hear it, Vicki, I really am. I'm sorry about everything that happened to you, but I'm happy you're healing."

Here's what I didn't say:

The failure of the military and our government to hold those men accountable is unacceptable. And though your victories were critical, they are small victories in the face of massive systemic failures. The systemic corruption revealed by the crimes against you is abhorrent, shameful, and illegal. Men must be made to pay for their crimes.

But there was no way to say those things in that moment without undermining her process. It certainly wasn't the time for that.

"Thank you, thank you. I told my grandma I was going to school, and I'm going to go. I just have to get well. My old therapist, the one I saw when I first got back, she said I have major depressive disorder and am probably bipolar, something like that. I just hope I can overcome it."

"Vicki, first of all, you are well. I want you to know that your feelings are normal. You were traumatized. You were in horrific conditions, and your human response to those horrific conditions is normal."

She looked at me and seemed to be softening. Her breathing slowed as she rested in the chair.

"What's not normal, what's not healthy, is if those things happened and you didn't feel sad or angry. You're right, you do need to start to feel better so that you can be happy and fulfilled. That's all. You're not sick. You're not abnormal. You're a survivor who's doing amazing things to heal herself."

Vicki paused. Her eyes focused as she looked across the room, and then she nodded to herself as she considered the entirety of the situation.

"It's true," she said aloud, but to herself.

She grasped her left fist with her right and anchored her hands low over her pelvis. Then she looked up at me. "You know, Doc, I don't even know whose child it was." Her voice thinned to a plea as she cast her eyes down. "That's what happens when different people rape you." Her words landed heavily in the space between us. We let them be there in their hugeness, in their horror.

"How could that pastor tell *me* to forgive? They should all go to hell. But *I'm* the one sinning for not forgiving?" A solitary tear rolled from her eye, landing on the side of her right cheek before she swiped it away.

"I hear you. You did *nothing* wrong. The men who did this to you were wrong. These men are weak and pitiful. You know that people who do awful things are really suffering so deeply, so profoundly."

"Now *that* I agree with. My mom stole from me because she was suffering. It took me a long time, but I finally forgave her. I forgave her before I went off to war. I saw her for who she was and what she was going through, so I forgave her." I could see her easing back into her strength.

"Yeah, like your mom. What she did was not right. You

saw her pain and understood it. You forgave her. It doesn't excuse her actions. It doesn't say that it was okay for her to behave that way. It only says that you recognized her pain and suffering and wished her healing. You released it. How did it feel to do that?"

"I felt free. I went away and felt free."

Her voice deepened as she began to find grounding in contemplation.

I said, "And that's the only reason to forgive the souls of these men who did these monstrous things. They are as troubled as the acts they committed."

"I hear you, Doctor. I just don't know that I can ever get over this. I have to heal, as you say. But some days, when I actually think about it, honestly, I don't know that I can."

I racked my brain for something true, for something I told myself when life felt too hard and unfair, for what I had told myself before coming into work and seeing a full board of patients in the VA ER and ED directors who regularly didn't show up for their shifts despite that fact; for what I said when I thought back on my childhood, my divorce, and the fact that I was still single in Philadelphia, a city that is famously unwelcoming to people who weren't conceived within the city limits—and yet, I couldn't just pick up and move without feeling that I was running away.

"You remember Nelson Mandela?" I asked her.

"Of course."

"What a loss for all of us that he passed away," I said,

frowning. "What a tremendous force for good, one that has now crossed over."

"I know; he was amazing," Vicki said, brightening.

"So, you remember what he went through? He fought to overcome institutionalized racism in his own government, and he was imprisoned for it. He was sent to prison for almost thirty years. Clearly, that's an abuse in and of itself, and he survived even more abuse while in prison. But he emerged to summon love, forgiveness, and compassion to literally change the world, therein healing himself and many millions of other people. His legacy speaks to what we human beings can withstand. What they did to you was wrong, Vicki. What they did to Mandela was wrong. So many things that happen to us are *not* right, are *not* okay. And we can survive and heal and use that to be stronger and shape our lives and the lives of others in wonderful, powerful, healing ways, should we choose to do so. Honestly, that's the reason to forgive. Just like with your mom: In your own time, you forgave her to free yourself. You forgave her to heal yourself. In your strength, in your courage, in your self-love, others are healed. That's all. All in time."

"I like that, Dr. Harper. I like that a lot. I really want to do that. That's why I'm here. That's why I'm going to school. My new squad is helping me. My new therapist is helping me, too."

"Most important, you're helping yourself. *You* are doing all of this."

Hearing that, she glowed with pride. "Yes, I am."

"Yes, you are. Go forth and be Mandela!" I joined my hands in front of my heart as if to say *Namaste*—a force of habit by that point.

She smiled. "Yes! That's why I'm here!"

"That's right, you're doin' it!" We laughed deep soul laughs together. For the first time, the room was buoyant. I forgot that I was late for sign-out. I forgot that I was in the psychiatric ER.

"Well, my dear, I've gotta go back to the medical side. My day here is done. All the best to you. One day, come back and tell me your stories of happiness and contentment. Congratulations already on your brand-new life."

"Thank you. I promise I will. You know what? I haven't ever talked to anyone like that. I've never told the whole story. I didn't know that would happen today. Feels so good to get it out. To let it go!"

She emanated a softening, a radiance that made her appear ten years younger than when she first came in. "Wow," I said. "You're okay and safe and your energy is lighter, too. You even look brighter."

"Thank you, Doctor. God bless you."

"Thank you and God bless you and us all. We all need it." I shared one last smile with her, then turned to open the curtain and walk away.

The night psychiatric nurse, Pat, approached. "What are you still doing over here? Didn't your shift end an hour ago?"

"Yeah, I have to skedaddle."

"What the heck happened just now? You miss your calling, Doc?"

"Huh?" I asked, but I knew he had heard. The unit was small, with no doors except those for the bathroom, the psychiatrist's office, and the social work office, so there was no privacy. You could hear every word from the patient rooms, every word at the nurses' desk.

"Your calling as a shrink!" he replied.

I laughed. "Have a great night, guys. I'll see y'all again in a couple of days."

I swiped my ID card at the exit to liberate myself from the unit.

Vicki and I had both crossed thresholds that day. We had both braced ourselves and covered our heads as the walls of our glass houses had shattered around us. We had trod mindfully over the shards and escaped with nonfatal wounds to a new freedom, a new clarity, a new resolve. As I passed the full tracking board and the poorly staffed ER, I recalled that I still had five or six notes to complete before signing out, which meant I'd be there for another twenty minutes. But that was all right: I felt lighter and brighter, too. Vicki's strength was a true testament to human mettle, a beacon.

I thought back on the things that had been upsetting me just an hour before—whether or not to move, the dismal social scene in Philly, the administrative problems in the hospital that were consistently infuriating, and most of all, the bizarre hospital politics that had shot down my proposal to start a complementary medical center at the VA to treat the chronic effects of trauma such as pain, depression, and anxiety. The center would have been modeled after centers of excellence at other VA hospitals in the country. Despite my having presented data from those hospitals and from the U.S. military showing improved outcomes from complementary treatments, treatments that lacked the detrimental side effects of the drugs comprising the bulk of remedies offered at our site, the proposal was repeatedly rejected without any specific reason. At one point, the vague explanation given was that there was some guy at the Philadelphia VA who did pain management, so if anyone should start such a clinic, it should be him—the same guy who *hadn't* started one in over a decade.

The members of CAM, the Complementary and Alternative Medicine Interest Group (comprising committed internal medicine physicians, social workers, and psychiatrists who met monthly to discuss ways to safely improve the lives of veterans), had tried to warn me. They had tried for years to get such a center off the ground, but there had always been a barrier. One month, the hospital administration told them there was no space for it; another month, there was no funding; then, the next year, it just wasn't the right time. Unable to effect change, one by one, the members of the group had left the Philadelphia VA. As for my center, its creation wasn't foreseeable in any near decade, and unlike the CAM group, I was given no reason for this, so I could not prepare a counter pitch. The better part of valor was to take all of it as a sign from the universe that I should try something else.

Reflecting on my conversation with Vicki, I realized that none of my concerns was truly debilitating. I would get home eventually, and this would have been a very good day, a very good day in a very blessed life.

Standing in my kitchen that evening, as the steam welled up from my caramel tea, I was suffused with the lessons I'd learned from Victoria Honor and the reminder that, whether on the mat or off, we always have the choice to start again, to bind again exquisitely.

EIGHT

Joshua: Under Contract

IT WAS EARLY—well before 6 a.m. and still dark. To spend the entire day working and then leave the hospital in this same darkness was always disorienting, but I preferred arriving early to running in late to the doctors' lounge, locs flying, ID swinging, after the unofficial ten-minute late mark. Anything up to ten minutes late was moderately irritating to people but not entirely unreasonable. That nine-plus-minute allowance was there in case we got caught behind a bus or were detoured by a freak accident. Today I didn't need that buffer; instead, I walked slowly from the parking lot to the hospital and settled into the ER staff lounge to eat my breakfast of Greek yogurt with almonds and blueberries as I sipped myself awake with coffee.

The bonus in arriving early was that there was time to get caught up reading the latest medical journal issue. The hospital was still quiet—no footsteps; no rolling wheelchairs; no voices asking directions to a room; no police officer escorting a belligerent patient. The only sound was the night shift's percolating coffeemaker, whose smoky aroma was wafting me alert. Sitting in the staff lounge, I looked up at the clock: 5:45 a.m.

Today will be a good day, I silently affirmed. Somewhere between shifts, I'd have to figure out the rest of my life. But not right now.

I had been practicing medicine long enough to know that wellness was much more than anything we prescribe from a bottle. If we humans were to expand our definition of healing, there could actually be a great deal more of it. For the time being, my complementary medicine center idea had crashed and burned. I had been so committed to this path that when I was turned down, I had even looked into starting a center outside the VA. After taking a number of courses through the Philadelphia Small Business Administration, and after months of meeting with my mentor from the SBA, and with many local professionals, I had learned that the market in Philadelphia would make it nearly impossible to earn a living with such a business for any time in the near future; it just wouldn't be feasible unless I wanted to continue to work full time clinically and then use the alternative medicine business as an extremely expensive and time-consuming hobby.

But even with that disappointment, my career was faring better than my personal life. I was several years past my divorce and several years past an extremely brief (but still too long, at several months) and dismal interlude of online dating. I was still single. But there was an even more depressing truth: I had fallen into an impossible love. Just the week before, I had told Colin, the cop I was seeing, not to contact me again. His divorce was proving to be more difficult than he had initially presented to me, and far more difficult than he had allowed himself to believe. It was taking all but a military extraction for him to sever ties from the person who had stolen his phone, hacked his online accounts to steal data and post false information on him, stalked him, physically assaulted him, and mused about fabricating a disturbance at his work so he would lose his job. Oh, and then there were her repeated threats to set his property on fire. There was still time for her to make good on those last two threats, regarding the career assassination and the arson. Colin's ex had promised him that "the only thing I want is for you to suffer." If what Colin had told me and what I had observed were accurate, this seemed to be the only completely honest statement she had uttered in her life.

Strange how police officers frequently find the wackadoos. I suppose it's just like ER physicians, psychiatrists, social workers, and all of us in the helping fields: We all nurse that same Achilles' heel of cleaving to the damaged. What a critical life lesson: to learn to distinguish enabling from helping, codependence from love, attachment to reenacting the grief of childhood loss from allowing for the sweetness of self-determination.

To go into detail about my relationship with Colin would

certainly bore even the most sympathetic reader. Suffice it to say, there was a lot about it that I appreciated. For example, it was more fun preparing dinner together than dining out in a fancy restaurant. Colin taught me how to cook the perfect stovetop steak and a reliably fluffy omelet (although, I still prefer to be the sous chef or, even better, official taste-tester for these types of culinary pursuits). While one of my all-time favorite solo excursions is devouring a weekday matinee at the local independent movie theater, the 1 p.m. film experience couldn't hold a candle to the two of us cuddling up in front of HBO with kettle corn and tea. There's no point in going into detail about all that because it's the typical cheese.

What was singular was the connection—that was the stuff. When he and I met, I was half-hurrying to work—I say "half" because traffic was moving well that day, which was never guaranteed in Center City, so I had time to enjoy the beautiful weather for a couple more minutes before getting into my car. Colin, in plainclothes, greeted me in the parking lot by saying I looked focused. He followed it up with "Are you working hard or hardly working?" I hadn't paid him any attention until those words fell from his mouth. That's when I looked up at him. There was no way I could contain my eruption of laughter following his hilariously terrible pickup line. Relieved at my willingness to engage despite his pitiful approach, he laughed, too, then stumbled backward. It was strange because he didn't trip; there was nothing on the pavement. He just fell backward, then caught himself with an opportune step. We stood there staring at each other with an uncanny recognition. I squinted, then finally broke the stare by stating that I had to run to work, knowing the real reason for my hurrying off was that the prolonged gaze with a stranger felt inappropriate, although the description of "stranger" didn't seem to fit him. From the beginning, we could talk about the meaning of faith until three in the morning. How, just by seeing the crinkle in my brow or hearing a three-second pause in my speech, he could read my mind. How, once, at 2 a.m., I woke up from a deep sleep feeling him, across town, thinking about me. I had been comfortable in bed—it wasn't too hot or cold; I didn't have to use the bathroom; there was no nightmare or particular issue—I just woke up with this sense. I looked at my phone to see that there was no voice mail message, no missed call, no text. I replaced the phone on the end table, fluffed my pillow, then rolled over for round two of sleep. That's when the phone rang, and it was him.

Then he changed—the way desperate people sometimes change; the way hurt people can change. They don't change from who they are, but they reveal what is deep inside. Yes, he was tired from divorcing a woman who fought dirty, but his bigger battle was within himself. He was angry that he had found himself with such a person in the first place. The trauma he was experiencing triggered old wounds of being abandoned by a mother who frequently left him in the care of an uncle who, when Colin was a little boy, beat him like a man. No one rescued him then. This same mother was verbally aggressive with him to this day; it was her well-worn coping mechanism. So, he had grown up to replicate his childhood abuse by finding toxic relationships that would remind him of his past, because he hadn't yet resolved those wounds. Now he was fighting to rescue himself from all of it. He was in crisis, and this deserved sympathy.

But wounded animals can turn vicious as they fight for their lives. He became irritable, withdrawn, and unkind. It wouldn't be fair to say he stayed that way. He didn't—he got worse. He became someone I couldn't like in a casual way, much less love in a romantic one. As I wondered which aspect of Colin would prevail in the end, and what that would be like, I realized that the most sensible question I should be asking myself was: What part of my unresolved wounds bonded with his trauma?

Then I saw it. His collapsing in times of crisis was my mother. His lashing out from a place of core fear was my father. His spiraling denial and now codependence was them both. Colin and my shadow selves reenacted familiar patterns from our common pasts. The experience with him reminded me that I had *consciously* chosen a different pattern for myself long before, so I needed to choose an action consistent with that decision. Furthermore, I wasn't his ex, his uncle, his mother, or his wounded inner child. But if I stayed through that period, I would have been all of them, because in the midst of his battle, he couldn't tell whom he was fighting anymore.

Timing can make or break the best of us, and for reasons that may be yet to be revealed. When I left him, which, unlike my divorce, took not only a series of conversations but eventually my quietly blocking him on every platform because there are, after all, only so many times it is reasonable to have the same conversation, he told me that he knew he would never have a relationship with this depth of love again in his life. We both knew that was true. He let me know, too, that he would come back for me, to see if he could make it right when he could make it right. If he could reach me in time, before life made his return impossible, before he heard of my living in some faraway place or with another man in another life, I knew that he would try. But life evolves.

"This lifetime or the next, my love, we'll reunite," I told him. "This lifetime or the next." I meant it at the time. And while Colin was sold on neither reincarnation nor the delayed gratification of next-life reunification, he knew that what I said somehow rang true. It still makes me smile that though it was at times difficult for him to hear, he always believed everything I said.

I got it, too, how good people can lose their way during life transitions. How they can behave in self-destructive ways until they master another pattern—should they ever choose another pattern. In my life, I chose a different pattern from the one I was born into, so I would not replay my past trauma with anyone. It was worth creating good with the right person at the right time. *I* am worth being healthy with a person who also chooses health.

So, I blessed him and walked away. While I felt a forever

connection with him even when I left, I knew that in time this would change. I couldn't predict when the sight of fresh herbs wouldn't make me think of the garden he said he'd plant for me; or when I'd stop waking up mid-REM sleep in a panic, knowing that somewhere he was staring at his phone and trying not to call. But I knew that someday, in a future I could feel but not yet see, I wouldn't want him back. It didn't matter where I lived or whether I was with someone else or alone: I knew myself well enough to know that when I leave, I leave for better and I leave for good. First comes the physical separation; the emotional disentanglement follows in time.

Life had to get easier. There had to be a day, and soon, when I could coast for a little while. I was exhausted.

Then I autocorrected to remind myself of a more effective affirmation: Today *is* a good day, I thought. (I breathed it in.) Today is a day of blessings and gratitude. (I breathed it out.)

I sipped my favorite coffee, Fair Trade French Roast, that I had ground fresh and hand-poured this morning, and kissed with coconut sugar and cream. Today *is* a lucky day. This moment *is* a blessing.

I folded up my half-read medical journal and headed over to the ER.

As I rounded the corner, I peeked at the tracking board. Six patients slated for admission, three patients up for discharge. One of the dedicated night physicians, Marlee, was just wrapping up her shift. She worked at the VA on a per diem basis, so we saw her only rarely. Marlee was also leaving the VA soon. (With the constant turnover of staff in the department, we were used to having colleagues come and go.)

"Hello, Marlee. How was the night?" I asked.

"Girl, same ol' same ol'!" I never could figure out how Marlee did it. Every time I saw her after a night shift, she looked as bright-eyed and dewy and hopeful as if she'd just walked in to work. The chaos of the shift never left one hair out of place in her smooth ponytail. Her skin was *still* so fresh and well hydrated—presumably from the strawberry-infused water she always brought with her. She was a wonder to behold.

"You know this place really robs you of momentum," she added. "It's just so hard to get things *done* here. Four patients waiting for admission since yesterday—how is that okay? All the while, I'm here alone trying to see new patients while managing patients who are already admitted. It's not right for anyone."

I nodded. "I know. Always the same. We tell the powers that be," I said, making air quotes around "powers." "But for—"

"Nothing!" she interjected.

"Oh, Marlee." I sighed, smiling at her. "Maybe it'll get better soon. You know we're supposed to get some new administrators in the hospital. Maybe they won't abuse the staff, and folks will actually stick around. Who knows? Maybe, instead of creating fraudulent logs of hours worked to milk the system, the leaders will actually work to improve the care of veterans. We might even get enough provider coverage in the hospital . . . So maybe . . ."

Marlee gave me a sideways glance. "Michele, you keep believing! You go right ahead and keep on believing those nice thoughts!" Then she joined me in the only thing we could control: laughter.

She was right. As emergency medicine doctors, we commit ourselves to evaluating patients who come in "sick" before their root illness is known. We assess these patients to figure out if they are acutely ill, and then we determine treatment plans to address their individual needs. We do not do the work of the specialty teams who narrow their vision to one organ, we do not do the work of primary care providers who coordinate five different services to work up a tumor over the next two months and chase minor abnormalities in a patient's lab work for weeks. We are the ones who help people right now. We determine what is critical, what has to be addressed immediately, and then we address those critical issues before we send patients either off into the world, where they can manage it themselves; or to the hospital, where others will help them manage it for a time.

That is the understanding, the agreement, the contract that we emergency medicine physicians have with the patients, the hospital, our colleagues, and ourselves. When that contract is violated, it is a painful breach. Now, in an ER with so many patients boarding, in a department with a policy that the ER staff is to care for all boarding patients so that the ER physician now adds to her workload the duties of the other specialists as well as the general medicine teams until the patients are transported from the department to their hospital beds—despite this being in violation of VA policies and procedures, despite all the studies showing that admitted patients boarding in the ER have increased adverse outcomes—that contract *had* been violated.

So, I fell back to my contract with myself: First, do no harm; then heal.

No new patients had come into the department yet. It was a perfect time to scroll through the list of boarding patients to make sure nothing had been missed and nothing was still due.

Ms. Craig, who had been admitted last year for chest pain and had a history of a positive cardiac catheterization, which showed evidence of significant heart disease, was due for her second blood draw for her troponin level, to look for evidence of a heart attack.

Mr. Hornsby would need his third dose of antibiotics in three hours, for his cellulitis.

Ms. Grant had been admitted for renal failure and a urinary tract infection. The ceftriaxone she received would give her twenty-four hours of antibiotic coverage. We hoped she'd get a bed within six hours, so the next dose could be ordered by her admitting team.

Mr. Khan's blood pressure was stable after the seven doses of antihypertensive medication the last two shifts had given him.

Ms. Chen was comfortable and waiting for a bed for her lower GI bleed workup, with a plan for gastroenterology to scope her today.

Mr. Clements was waiting for a bed and workup on the source of his cancer and for pain control.

The four patients on the psychiatric side of the emergency department were all well and waiting for final disposition by the psychiatrist.

After reviewing all patient information, entering orders, and updating my patient list, I was caught up, with no new patients in the waiting room.

Nurse Sean pulled up a chair next to mine. "So, where's the next trip?" I asked him.

Sean and I had worked together years ago, at Andrew Johnson. Although he was probably twenty years my senior, our lives seemed to parallel. Back when he was leaving his marriage to be with the woman it made sense for him to marry, and I had freshly completed my divorce from the man I thought I was supposed to marry, we were both working in administrative positions. I was new to the role, and he was a seasoned veteran. Now, several years later, we had met again, in new phases of life. I had left academic medicine and administrative work to resume the clinical work I cared most about.

Sean was Irish American, with more rust-colored hair sprouting from the V-neck of his scrub top than on his head. Thanks to his wife's Sierra Leonean heritage, he had the distinction of being the best Irish cook of West African cuisine in all Philadelphia. He had given up his lifetime of administrative work for a per diem gig that allowed him to have the schedule of his choice, so he could travel with the woman he had anointed his "queen." It is no exaggeration to say that every several weeks, the two were on their way somewhere: Martinique, Niagara Falls, Hawaii, Tennessee. Their life together was entirely intentional and, in that way, entirely inspiring.

"Next we go to Paris," Sean said, leaning back in the chair, arms folded behind his head and feet propped up on a stool. Before the next five patients registered to be seen, he and I had time to catch up on their plans to visit the Louvre and his desire to see General Patton's grave.

Ten patients and two and a half hours later, the second attending should have arrived. I looked at the board and noticed that none of my patients from the night shift had been assigned to admitting physicians. One patient was waiting to be seen by my colleague—whenever he deigned to show up for his shift. Three patients were being sent to the ER for evaluation from outpatient clinics—this despite our being "on diversion," that is, unable to accept transfers from other facilities due to our not having the capacity to care for them. One of those outpatients had even been called in from home. Four other patients were in the waiting room about to come into the ER; and now five patients were waiting for admission. The one psychiatric patient who was to go home that morning was now sober from his alcohol intoxication, but he was confused. The nurse called me to assess him; he knew only his name but had no idea of the date, place, or situation. Reviewing his records, I could tell that this was not the baseline for this otherwise healthy middle-aged white man. I started his medical workup and then made a string of phone calls to find out when the boarding patients would get inpatient beds and teams to manage their care.

Gloria, the trusty and hardworking bed coordinator, informed me that not only were there no beds available, but there were "negative beds."

"What do you mean by *negative* beds?" I asked.

"I mean the OR has a full schedule, and I have no place to put all the post-op patients, nowhere to put the ER patients waiting for admission, and there are no discharges planned. *Negative* beds."

"And it's only nine a.m.," we said in unison.

"Awesome," I said. "Well, Gloria, please keep me posted."

"Yeah, I'm working on it. I'm going up to the floors now to tell the docs to get people moving."

I reached out to the ER medical director, leaving a voice mail, text, and email asking for the higher-ups to mobilize hospital beds and to continue our diversion status from transfers from other hospitals in light of this Monday morning madness. As was typical of the ER leadership in this institution, there was no answer, no return message, no help.

I asked myself: How much inpatient medicine could I safely perform while still attending to the care of the steady stream of brand-new ER patients? I knew that the new ER patients had to be seen. Could I safely leave those boarding patients to linger in the ER unattended? Even if it was safe to do so, was it ethical?

To the layperson, these may sound like silly questions, but would you expect an auto mechanic with a full schedule to stay on task with each new vehicle and at the same time help each client get directions home, coordinate vehicle pickup and child care, and schedule follow-up appointments? Of course not. Yes, these details fall under the category of "it's not my job," but that's what doctors are often called to do, and it's what makes it impossible for us to excel at what is actually our job. In emergency medicine, as in the case of the over-worked mechanic, working outside one's prescribed duties makes the work dangerous. All this, of course, doesn't answer the most important question I was forced to answer: How many of the shortcomings of this modern health care system was I willing to put up with? Or, perhaps better, would my healing mission be better served in other ways?

So, at 9:40 a.m., with a growing backlog of patients and still no sign of the second attending physician, I wondered what to do. First, I knew, was to do no harm: My patients were all stable, with the exception of the man with the newly altered mental state. I would evaluate him first and, if necessary, order additional labs, an EKG, a head CT, and vitamins, as he was a known alcoholic and could have a vitamin deficiency that put him at risk for permanent brain damage.

Next, I would see any new patients who were waiting.

Then, to heal: I would initiate any plans I anticipated the

inpatient teams would have for the boarding patients who had been waiting the longest in the ER. While adding this to my list of tasks would make my work exponentially harder, it wasn't the patients' fault they were still stuck in the ER.

The best way to start, I thought, was to get another cup of coffee and then dive in.

I called Cardiology to come see the patient with chest pain, and I called GI to see my GIB (gastrointestinal bleed) patient. Both services were very confused as to why they were getting a call from me, rather than the inpatient teams, and they asked if the admitting physicians could call for the consultations once the patients were on their floors, as this was standard hospital procedure. I explained that I, too, was confused by the chronic delays in patient care in the hospital, and that I was trying to expedite these patients getting care while they waited in limbo. The departments agreed to see the patients in the ER. Similar calls followed, to Neurology and the Echocardiography Lab, and the people there were similarly accommodating.

Next, I had to decide what to do with Mr. Clements. The notes from the last two attending physicians indicated that he was being admitted for pain control and a metastatic cancer workup. He had received one dose of pain medication since last night, and his vitals were normal. I had just passed his room and saw a well-dressed, slender man walking around, speaking calmly and comfortably on the phone—not the picture of a pain-control admission. A CT of his abdomen had revealed scattered swollen lymph nodes "too numerous to quantify," as the report read.

"Dr. Harper," Nurse Carissa called. "I just put a young guy in Room Six. He only has a psych history of some depression and anxiety, but he comes in today with fever, tachycardia in the one-thirties, infection from shooting drugs."

Putting my phone calls and Mr. Clements on hold again, I followed Carissa directly to Room 6.

"Good morning, Mr. Spano," I said.

He was seated on the stretcher, looking contained and anxious. I turned to the man standing at his side, who appeared to be a carbon copy of him. "Hello. Are you two related? You must be. You look exactly alike."

"Yeah, I'm his brother."

I turned back to the patient. "What brings you in today?"

"An infection, ma'am."

He had long brown hair, olive skin, and the stocky build of an ex-athlete. It was clear that before the depression and before the drugs, he had been an attractive young man. He was only twenty-nine, but with the pallid skin of a man thirty years his senior.

He grimaced as he bent his right leg, pointing to a sausage-like calf with puffy, flaking black skin that looked like charcoal. As he looked at his leg, tears rolled down his cheeks, and he wept out loud.

"How did this happen?" I asked him.

"Ma'am, I'm not gonna lie. I shot up crack. There might have been some heroin in there, too. I don't know."

"Hmmm," I said, nodding as his shoulders shook under his sobs. "This is a very serious infection. We'll need to—"

"What? What do you mean? Why do you say that?" he yelled.

"Well, you have a fever and—"

"A fever?" he interrupted again, his face twisting in agony. He covered his mouth as he whimpered and shook his head. "I didn't have a fever before!"

I recoiled from him. It might have been the volume of his exclamations or maybe the drama unfolding before me that caused me to cringe.

"As I was saying, you have a fever here, and your heart rate is very fast. Those two things tell us your infection is significant. Do you have pain?"

"Pain? I have tremendous pain—one hundred out of ten!"

"Okay, what we'll need to do is check your blood, get X-rays, and give you antibiotics and IV fluid. I'll also give you medicine for fever and pain while we sort everything out. Because your infection looks quite serious, I'll need to speak to a surgeon, in case you need an operation to fix this. No matter what, I'll have to keep you in the hospital, because you'll need to be continued on intravenous antibiotics for a couple of days or so."

"Oh, no!" he shrieked, in a voice much higher than one might guess his two-hundred-pound frame would be able to produce. "Am I going to die from this? Could I die from this?"

I spoke slowly, my voice soft, my tone deliberate, as I tried to tamp down his frenzy and instill clear boundaries.

"It's too early to say. You have a very serious infection. People can die from infections like this. Most people with this are fine as long as we do everything to treat it well. That's what we're doing here today."

"Pull it together, dude!" his brother interrupted, sounding intoxicated. He had a beard as scruffy as his voice and wore a black T-shirt that rolled over a loose stomach and soft silver athletic shorts.

His brother's words only seemed to add fuel to the fire of agony in Mr. Spano, who now began to weep inconsolably. "Oh my God," he whimpered, burying his face in his hands.

Carissa and I looked at each other and tried not to raise our eyebrows. His reactions were so far out of proportion to what was going on. Patients who are struck by cars or who receive new diagnoses of cancer demonstrate more composure than this young man was showing. Sure, he was ill, but the odds were that he would rapidly improve after a couple of days of intravenous antibiotics before switching over to antibiotic pills.

Carissa placed an IV in him and drew blood. I completed my physical exam. He was awake and alert throughout—no lethargy. His heart sounds were fast but regular, with no murmur. It seemed that his drug use hadn't damaged his heart. He had no rash. Good blood flow to his skin. His right leg was normal down to the shin. The area between the knee and the ankle was swollen but soft. While the leg was markedly swollen, red, and warm to the touch, his tenderness was greater than his physical exam suggested. When I pressed the tissue of his calf, I didn't feel the crackling that would have indicated necrotizing fasciitis, what the media had taken to calling "flesh-eating bacteria." The inner aspect of his calf had a necrotic abscess about the size of a silver dollar, though. I couldn't feel a collection of pus anywhere else, and yet, given the extent of his pain, and the swelling and tachycardia, I couldn't be sure there wasn't a deeper area of abscess or gas formation in the leg.

I explained to the patient and his brother that I was leaving the room to enter all his orders and call the surgeon. I informed them that this was time sensitive, so we needed to start his treatment quickly, but first I looked the patient squarely in the eye.

"Do you have any questions before I go?"

Mr. Spano shook his head, and I proceeded to leave. Just as I approached the door, his brother stopped me and asked, "How could this have happened?"

"Your brother injected drugs into his leg. That is the way this infection happened."

The contemptuous expression on his face upon receiving my answer was the same one I might have made after being awakened from a deep sleep by a phone call from a telemarketer.

Mr. Spano said nothing. Then he whimpered softly, "No, no, further questions. Thank you for helping me."

"You're welcome. I'll go get all those orders in for you," I said, turning to leave.

His brother stopped me again. "Can't we get him somewhere better? I'm sure there is a better hospital with better doctors to take care of this."

I paused before I spoke, narrowing my eyes as I felt the back of my throat constrict and my upper chest tighten. I knew there was no point in saying the first thing that came to mind: *How dare you?* Instead, I replied, "The treatment of this is very standard and is the same no matter if he's treated here or anywhere in the world. It would be the same if he were in Timbuktu, Yale New Haven Hospital, or the middle of a medical campground. It's all the same medicine."

"Okay, well, let's just do it, then," the brother said, as if granting me permission.

"Yeah," I said. Then I left, letting the curtain flap closed behind me.

My contract stipulated that I was to help this man, *to heal* him no matter what. I did not like him or his brother. I did not like that they were rude and histrionic. I did not like that they seemed not to take personal accountability for what was happening to them. I felt drained by the patient's hysteria and his brother's condescension and demands. But I was there to help.

I quickly entered the orders—monitor, fluids, medications, EKG, labs, cultures, X-rays, and ultrasound—then put a page out to General Surgery, who quickly called back and told me that extremity infection concerns were covered by the orthopedic service. I paged Orthopedic Surgery and waited, and waited. Finally, I called the hospital operator and asked her to notify the ultrasound tech on call, only to be told that there was no ultrasound tech on call this holi-day weekend, so we wouldn't be able to evaluate the dimen-sions of the abscess in that way. I was well aware that the orthopedic surgeon would need to know the size and depth of the abscess in addition to looking for deeper gas collections in the tissues to determine the appropriate treatment plan.

While I was working on behalf of the Spanos, the ER had been backing up with patients. There was still no answer from Orthopedics, so I picked up the phone again to page the on-call attending orthopedic surgeon myself. It was both a blessing and a curse that our surgical attendings were also faculty at the nearby teaching hospital. The blessing was that it meant more staff, both attending and resident physicians, to care for patients. The curse was that nine times out of ten, they called back angry and affronted be-cause, unlike in the community, academic faculty typically did not have the same incentives to build relationships as the private practice providers who welcomed our calls to be in-volved in patient care. But still, additional financial incen-tive or not, it always struck me as strange that a person on schedule to work in his chosen field should be angry when called to do the work he signed up to do.

As I waited, documenting the patient's condition on his chart, Nurse Jen showed up at my side and asked me to please speak with Mr. Clements.

Yes, I had meant to get back to Mr. Clements! "Sure thing, Jen. He's next on my list. I just have to speak to Orthopedics, and I'll be right in."

"Thank you, because he's asking for pain medication, but he looks fine. I think he really just wants to speak to a doctor."

"I'll be right there. Sorry 'bout the delay."

Fortunately, the orthopedic resident called back and said he would come to the ER after rounds and after seeing a patient at another hospital. Meanwhile, he requested a CT of Mr. Spano's leg, as there was no way to complete an ultrasound.

Finally, I headed to Room 18, to see Mr. Clements. As I approached his room, I saw a tall, lean man with long dreadlocks gathered into a trim ponytail grazing his waist. He appeared to be a remarkably youthful sixty-eight years old. With his hands resting resignedly in his linen pants pockets, he paced slow circles in his room, periodically stopping to look up at the TV screen in the corner. I walked to the room and knocked on the open door. I smiled and introduced myself. He extended his hand to shake and said, "I like your hair, Doctor," indicating my own tied-back dreads.

"Thank you. And yours as well," I said, smiling. "Mr. Clements—"

"Please, call me Joshua," he interjected.

"Joshua." I nodded, smiling at him. "I'm so sorry for all the delays. I understand you're waiting for a bed upstairs to find out why you have this lymph node swelling all over the place. I also understand you've had pain. Do you still have pain?"

"I do, Doc. The pain is coming back. It's not bad. It's not

like when I came in last night, but a little pain is coming back," he said, rubbing the front of his abdomen to indicate the location.

"Would you like more pain medication?" I offered.

"I've never been much into pills. It's just not the type of man I am, but yeah, today I'd like some."

"Of course. Let's chat about your CT findings also. The doctor on overnight was telling me you have a history of cancer, many years ago?" I asked.

"Yes, almost twenty years ago I had prostate cancer and two big tumors in my liver. I told them they could do surgery to cut them out. They wanted me to do chemo and radiation, too. The doctors kept pressuring me about that, but I didn't do it, Doctor. I just couldn't. So many people told me I was crazy, but to me, those supposed cures just felt like poison. Instead, I took herbal supplements and ate healthy. I went on long walks and felt good. That's just my way, Dr. Harper. I prefer to keep things natural. I know it was a gamble no matter what I decided, but I've lived a healthy life and cleansed my body that way. Luckily, I've been fine ever since—well, until now. It's just that I had some pain in my belly last night, so I came in to have it checked out."

The CT findings indicated a malignancy.

This poor guy, I thought. There's a macabre medical maxim that says that the good people get the worst diseases. If a person is generous of spirit and comes in with a nagging abdominal discomfort the week after she runs a marathon, we'll discover she has stage-four ovarian cancer. The racist pedophile who drowns kittens on Sundays survives being struck by lightning and lung cancer as he chain-smokes into his nineties. I was almost certain—almost—that there was no truth to this rule, apart from it proffering an emotional cocoon for us to fold ourselves into during difficult conversations.

I never liked being the doctor in the ER who, after knowing a patient for mere moments, and with only the benefit of a CT report and no definitive result such as a tissue pathology, had to introduce the word *cancer* into the discussion. But I knew it was cancer. I knew, too, that he wanted to know. I sensed that this man preferred the truth served up straight because it honored his right to choose.

"I see, I see. Now, did the doctor last night tell you that whenever we see lymph nodes like this, we get concerned that it's from cancer somewhere?"

"Nah, she didn't really tell me. She was kinda talking around in circles about swelling and nodes, but she didn't say the word *cancer*. Honestly, she didn't have to say it. I know what these findings on a CT mean. So, what's happening now? What's next? Will I just stay in this room all day?"

"You know, Mr. Clements—Joshua—that's an excellent question. Right now there are no beds in the hospital, and it looks like there won't be any for a long time. Maybe not until later this evening or even tomorrow."

"Oh, Dr. Harper, I can't stay here. I'm a vegan, so I can't even eat hospital food. And I haven't eaten since yesterday afternoon."

He was correct. This was no place for this man to use up more of his life, lying between bleached sheets, in a room with no natural light and no plants, forced to decline a breakfast tray of processed meat and eggs.

"I'm sorry about that, about the delays and the food," I said, then paused. "Joshua, I have to be honest with you. In your case, you don't really need to be admitted to the hospital. A cancer workup is the kind of thing that is typically completed as an outpatient, and I really think you'll be more comfortable that way. Of course, we can continue with your admission to the hospital as well. I'll leave the choice to you. I'm just saying, why be cooped up here when you can be comfortable at home and outside in this beautiful weather? If you like, I can write you a prescription for pain medication to take at home, if needed, and I can call the oncology doctor now to make sure you're scheduled for an appointment where the evaluation can be finished. The decision is yours."

He was a man who wore freedom more handsomely than any confine, so this idea suited him well. "Please, please. That sounds so much better. I don't want to be cooped up here if it's not necessary."

"Let me just call the oncology doctor now and see what they say, in case there's any additional information they'll need before you go. Is that all right?"

He clasped his hands in front of his chest and bowed his head slightly as he looked at me. "Yes! You'll come back and let me know?"

"I'll let you know. I promise," I said, smiling.

The oncology doctor called back and requested that I order a couple more blood tests as part of the cancer workup, including a PSA level and a chest CT for cancer staging. Her office would take Mr. Clements's information and call him for an appointment within the week.

Mr. Clements, apparently relieved by this expedited evaluation, agreed to stay to complete these studies. He then called his family with updates and asked them to bring him food, since he would be with us a couple more hours.

As I finished placing these additional orders, the orthopedic doctor came over to let me know that he had seen Mr. Spano and drained his abscess at his bedside. He recommended that he be admitted to the Internal Medicine service for intravenous antibiotics, as we had discussed. He warned me, though, that Mr. Spano was refusing to stay.

"What?" I said, baffled. "You're kidding. He was just begging for us to save his life."

"Not kidding," he responded as he left the department.

I reviewed Mr. Spano's results. His vital signs were now normal, and his labs were reassuring. His CT showed a superficial abscess and soft tissue swelling, but no gas formation—more good news.

I hurried down the hallway to Mr. Spano's room. He was sitting in a chair, shoving his feet into his sneakers. His brother had apparently already left, and he was now alone in the room with Carissa, who was trying to explain to him how important it was for him to be admitted to the hospital as planned.

"Mr. Spano, what's going on?" I asked, pretending not to know anything about his newfound urgency to leave.

"I gotta get out of here," he snapped. "I have things to do. I can't just lie around here. I'm better now. I need to go."

"Mr. Spano, you're better because we gave you a lot of very strong medicine to treat you. You'll need more of that medication to ensure you continue to get better."

"Well, then I can just leave with this IV. Just give me the medicine and I'll inject myself, or I can get my family to do it. I have family members who are nurses and doctors."

"Mr. Spano, you cannot leave with the IV. Your leaving with this IV would be against every hospital policy everywhere."

"Well, then just give me pills," he said, tearing the IV out of his arm and throwing it to the ground. Blood dripped from his arm onto the floor, and he snatched a piece of gauze off the medicine cart next to him, held it to his arm, and then threw it to the floor next to the IV he had already discarded. He stooped down to tie his shoelaces.

"If you must leave, I'll certainly write you a prescription for antibiotic pills to take at home, but Mr. Spano, remember when you came in just a couple of hours ago? Remember when you sat on that stretcher crying and begging us to save your life? Remember how I told you that you have an infection that could kill you?"

His hands stopped mid-bow on the left laces. For a moment he looked at me, and seemed to follow my point reluctantly. He nodded.

"Well, that is still the case. You still need that medication. You could still get very sick and perhaps die if you leave now without adequate treatment."

"Listen, there are other things I have to do," he said, bending over to complete the last lace. He stood up again and walked over to the side table to collect his jacket and phone. "I can't just sit here all day and night in a hospital. I have to finish paperwork for a job interview. I have a court hearing for custody of my son next week."

"If all goes well, you'll be out of the hospital within a couple of days," I told him. "That won't conflict with court next week. As far as paperwork, isn't there a way you could complete it here?"

"Listen, I just have too much to do, so I'm leaving," he said.

After he left, Carissa and I looked at the trash on the floor and the trail of blood.

"What a waste," Carissa said, as she kicked the trash into a pile and threw a chuck (a large medical napkin with a surface to soak up liquids) over the blood. "I knew he was gonna do that from the very beginning. What a complete and utter waste of time."

Mr. Spano had left without his prescription for antibiotics, without the dressing changes for his leg, without his discharge instructions, and without follow-up appointments.

I walked back to my station to scribble out some notes stating that Mr. Spano had left against medical advice. I forwarded the notes to his primary care provider and to Orthopedics, hoping that one or both services would try to contact him to make sure he was healing well.

Within ninety minutes, a very patient Joshua Clements would also get to go home. Radiology called again, providing a reading of his chest CT that was much like the CT of his abdomen: "Nodules too numerous to count." While the normal range for prostate-specific antigen is around 4, his level was over 200. I called Urology, who took his information for a walk-in appointment in four days to discuss what was certain to be a widely metastatic prostate cancer.

I called back the oncology service, who appreciated the follow-up and reported that someone would call Mr. Clements later that day to set up an appointment. Then I went back to his room to find him flanked by a fortysomething couple; the man's face was almost identical to his. The spirit in the room was aloft with laughter.

"Hello, everyone. I'm Dr. Harper. I'm back to give you the most recent results before you get on with your day."

"Dr. Harper, this is my son, Reid, and my daughter-in-law, Tracy," Mr. Clements announced, making his introductions.

"Hello," I said, greeting each of them. "So, Mr. Clements—"

"Joshua," he reminded me.

"Oh, yes, sorry. I keep doing that! Joshua, I have two more results for you. Your PSA level, the level for your prostate antigen, is super high. You probably remember talk of this from your last bout with prostate cancer."

"Yes, yes, I do."

"Also, the CT of your chest shows the same thing as your abdomen: numerous nodules everywhere. The combination of all this information suggests that this is all coming from the prostate cancer we were discussing earlier."

"I figured, Dr. Harper. I figured it. Wow," he said, looking at his children. "Wow, I feel fine!" He placed his hands on his chest and took deep, ample breaths as his hands expanded with each inhalation and contracted with each exhalation. "They're all over my chest, but I'm breathing fine." He looked at his children and continued to drink in the air. Lowering his hands to his lap, he said, "You know, Doctor, I'm not afraid. I'm just not. I've had a really good life." And then he laughed—a joyous, relieved, contented laugh.

His son looked at him and then at me. "You know, he's right. This old man has had quite a run," he said, chuckling. "Now I have to run around behind him like I'm the dad!"

"Ah, then all is as it should be," I responded, joining them in laughter.

Joshua continued. "I eat clean, I live clean. After all this time, I can say I'm truly at peace with whatever is to be. I had cancer over twenty years ago, and they said I would die if I didn't let them irradiate my body or fill me up with chemicals. I didn't want that then and I don't want it now." He placed one hand on his chest and one on his abdomen. "So strange. I'm breathing fine. I'm feeling fine. I look fine, if I do say so myself!" He laughed aloud again. "But, no, I mean

I just really feel fine," he said, looking down at the body beneath his hands.

He inhaled for two counts and exhaled for four, looking down at his feet at the edge of the bed. Switching his attention to me, he smiled and repeated, "You know, I'm just not afraid. I'll go to those appointments, Dr. Harper, just so I know what exactly is going on. I won't do chemicals or radiation, but I'll get my diagnosis, then leave it be and feel this good for as long as I can."

His son and daughter-in-law looked at him, full of courageous love. In that moment, there was no doubt in my mind that this was the most peaceful room in the hospital, perhaps in all of Philadelphia. I wanted to stand there longer just to be with his presence. I wanted to exhale all my anxiety over the uncertainty of life and breathe in Joshua's absolute faith in the universe, his absolute love for his body regardless of its tumors, his absolute comfort in his own skin.

"Joshua, the oncology team will call you later today to schedule your appointment. I've already spoken to the urology team, and they want you to return for your appointment Friday morning at nine a.m. Will that work for you?"

He nodded.

I continued: "Of course, I'll write you prescriptions for pain and nausea medications, should you need them. Do you all have any more questions for me now?" I asked.

His children shook their heads. Joshua got up off the stretcher and put out his arms to signal a hug.

I felt my back stiffen—a reflex. We emergency room doctors don't get too close to patients. It could be a fear of bedbugs, contaminated blood, or maybe the sacred integrity of the boundary between doctor and patient, or even just a fear of getting too close to people we hand off to others. In the split second between his extending his arms and my lumbar muscle contraction, I considered the unwritten rule of maintaining at least a gloved hand's distance from patients at all times. In the second before his warm embrace and his kiss on my cheek, I decided that sometimes these boundaries are more effective at keeping us caged in rather than at keeping others out.

"Sis, I want to thank you for making me feel like a human being through all this."

"My pleasure. All the best to you all. All the best on this journey."

As Joshua and his family gathered his belongings, I returned to my station and wrote up the discharge paperwork for him and then checked the tracking board. I needed to follow up with my new patients from that morning and the ones who remained from the night before. Luckily, two of them had magically received beds. My colleague had finally arrived and picked up five patients—out of guilt, I was sure. I signed up for one of the remaining—a seventy-year-old man with chest pain and normal vitals who was currently pain-free and had a normal EKG. I put in all the typical orders, which would save time and buy me a solid forty minutes to catch up on the work from earlier.

It was a good time to make a quick coffee run. I needed

some form of caffeine to be able to do my work, but I needed the glimmer of sun and fresh air the ten-minute walk to Wawa would provide even more.

Later that evening, at home, I poured myself a glass of Côtes du Rhône and settled in to eat dinner, a healthy comfort meal I deserved. I was glad that I had treated myself to flowers two days before. Right then, there was nothing in the world better than sunflowers, peonies, and roses as the backdrop to my meal.

I contemplated my time with Mr. Spano and Joshua. I marveled that Mr. Spano, who, once he'd learned that he wasn't going to die that afternoon, had found the prospect of remaining in the hospital so unsettling that he had preferred to hobble out on a bloated red leg and risk dying a few days later, although he wasn't yet thirty. I wondered what it must have felt like for him, without the haze of intoxication, to blur the relationship between himself and the truth. What was so terrible to face that death would be preferable? How might his inner contract read that he would be consumed with such a compulsion?

I am not healthy and cannot commit to healing. I am not strong enough to heal. I am fearful, so I must run. I am not worth fighting for. I am not worth healing for. I cannot endure the pain of facing my life. Because I am afraid I cannot be here sober; besides, I cannot be helped. I do not love myself enough to take care of myself. I do not love myself enough to allow you to take care of me. I do not deserve wellness, so I return to what I deserve.

What struck me powerfully was that Mr. Spano had honored every word of his inner contract. (Like everyone, he had this right of self-determination.) We do this when we select the partner who confirms our feelings of unworthiness, when we pick the job that pays us less than we deserve. It is all the same. It is all part of that contract that even if we didn't write it for ourselves, we certainly co-signed.

I wondered, too, about my contract with myself. I wondered why the behavior of this self-hating man would rock me for even a second. I thought about how I needed to love myself enough to allow others to fulfill their contracts with themselves, be it Mr. Spano, my ex-husband, my father, my mother, Colin, the hospital administrators, or anyone else. Mr. Spano's contract demanded that he act in ways that were dismissive of my attempts to help him. A human being can never treat another person better than he treats himself. So, if he says things that are disrespectful, this is his contract. His contract has nothing to do with mine unless I allow it to—unless I uncover a clause, in minuscule print on page 5, a clause that I overlooked, that stipulates my need to be validated by the Mr. Spanos of the world in order to feel okay about myself. He was kind enough to prompt me to review that section again, to edit out that portion for good. In that way, he was an angel of the shift.

My forehead throbbed. Each pulsation pounded against the affirmation regarding the good day I was supposed to have had.

Then again, many events don't unfold the way we think

they are "supposed to." Leaving Colin had felt like an amputation, an amputation of the love we used to have and the love of the child he said we were destined to have. Colin had even named him. When I told him I knew that my destiny was to have a girl, he laughed and said, "No, dear. I only make boys." So, I had lost two boys that day: Colin and the son he imagined we would have, a familiar loss that echoed the ghosts of Nella and August but was magnitudes more painful the second time around. I would get through this, too, no matter what. Over the next couple of weeks, I would set my mind back to the career stuff. It was strange to be balancing all this on the heels of my recent rebuilding. My foundation wasn't yet set, so I certainly didn't feel strong enough to weather this storm.

I had just listened to an interview with Astro Teller, the director of Google X, who explained that failure isn't making mistakes, it's not launching one project after another that fails. No, Teller defined failure as identifying that a course of action you've taken doesn't work, but proceeding with it *anyway*. So, I guessed that in my course-correcting, I actually *wasn't* failing repeatedly.

I felt myself breaking into a smile as I gazed out on my herb garden. A new reality seeped in: I would have to destroy it. The ladybugs I'd put there to take care of the aphid infestation had proved only a temporary fix; as expected, after they'd feasted, they'd flown away to explore other parts of Center City. The diluted cayenne pepper spray had failed as well. What I had was an herb garden overrun with insects.

I promised myself that I would get to it, and even considered that I'd start another organic garden in a week or two.

I considered the energy and love that had so peacefully radiated from Joshua. I considered what it must feel like to live free from fear and to connect so closely with bliss. He had lived the way he wanted to, on his own terms. When he was faced with cancer when he wasn't yet fifty, he had refused chemotherapy and radiation. This decision had been radical twenty years ago, when Western medicine was even more paternalistic than it is today and when complementary medicine had an even smaller platform. Even now, though I embraced the therapeutic benefits of healthful nutrition, physical fitness, acupuncture, aromatherapy, mindfulness, and meditation, and believed that living well with integrity imparts greater benefits than most of what can be dispensed in a pillbox, I couldn't know what decision I would make in those circumstances. I understood the compulsion most people had to wage the hardest war with the strongest drugs Big Pharma could fathom. I could imagine that refusing chemo and radiation might feel like a death sentence, especially with so many scientific articles, doctors, and hospitals touting their efficacy. These voices can be hard to ignore. I also know that a person's medical decisions are both arduous and deeply personal.

In Joshua's embrace, I had sensed a life well lived. Of course, I didn't know the details, but I felt a body that was strong and loving now. I felt a man who said, *No matter what, I will live this life on my terms. I will decide who I am and what is right for this body.* And I received this second boon of the day: the knowledge that I, too, could elect to live this way now, while (as far as I knew) I wasn't riddled with tumors, while my lungs still worked and my heart still beat. I could live this way now while I had sight and touch, while I could still learn from experience and maintain an open heart and mind, and could share this gift with others. Some of us do this: When we select partners who live free, when we choose work that is a calling, when we see life as an adventure—it's all the same contract.

The statuesque man with smooth, dark skin and the waist-length locs had offered me a gift: the power to choose what was most nurturing to me. Even if that choice challenged the zeitgeist, the power was mine. In his embrace were new green shoots: the choice to grow.

NINE

Paul: Murda, Murda

IN A LAST-DITCH EFFORT to stay alert for the final hours of my shift, I fully inhaled the moist summer air. I had walked out to the ambulance bay for a couple of minutes of twilight serenity. As I noted the first glow of tangerine clouds rolling over the smoky blue sky at the western end of the methadone clinic, I yawned and stretched my arms over my head. Today there was no man nodding asleep as he crossed the intersection, no circle of women ashing cigarettes over strollers holding sleeping infants clutching bags of barbeque potato chips. No, today the methadone clinic was closed, as were most businesses in the University City section of West Philadelphia on Sunday morning. Only the rare vehicle rolled by: buses transporting shift workers like me, trucks on their way to and from the highway. No pedestrians just yet. Presumably, both the walk-of-shamers and the faithful had not yet made their way out of the house.

After I reveled in a few more moments of tranquility, I took the long way back to the ER, walking out through the ambulance driveway and then making my way to the front entrance. I had told the nurses where I was, but I always felt guilty stepping even three feet away from the ER for more than a few minutes. Walking through the VA's automatic front doors, I saw not a soul except my favorite police officer, Charles, making his rounds. Throughout the year, without notice or apparent precipitating event, Charles delivered trays of turkey sandwiches with cranberry sauce to the ER. But the reason he was my favorite was because when he saw me, he always smiled as if he were being reunited with a long-lost friend. Now I returned Charles's wave with a grin indicating that I remembered our story, too.

With gratitude, I saw that the department was still sleepy. Near 5:30 a.m., I settled in to enjoy uninterrupted time to clear out the inboxes of two old email accounts, vestiges of times past. I had kept them open so I could use them for store mailings, utility bills, my student loan automatic payment reminder, and other notices I wanted to see only sporadically. I deleted the emails twenty at a time. Every once in a while, I stumbled upon something interesting: Martha Stewart's tips on the perfect summer sandwich; an email from the Oprah site on the twenty questions to ask yourself before getting married; the latest edition of *Shambhala Sun*, a bimonthly magazine that explores Buddhist topics.

I clicked on one of the links in *Shambhala Sun*: "No Big Deal: On Metta and Forgiveness," by Heidi Bourne. It discussed one woman's journey toward forgiveness as she explored loving-kindness (*Mettā*) for her abusive father during a *Mettā* practice retreat. Through exercises, she had touched the depths of pain that were buried in the pit of her belly. She faced the nausea and released the tears and simply let go. The article concluded with a phone call to her father, after an estrangement of more than a decade, which led to the following realization: "The experience was like talking to someone from my very distant past. He was still him, I was still me, and that was it. No big deal. And yet, it was everything."

Another confirmation of the synchronicity of life. That week, I had received a letter from my father through the VA mail at work. Not surprisingly, the letter had languished in a bin with other mail for the emergency department for more than six months before it was finally delivered to my medical director's office. My boss handed me a stack of mail consisting of a couple of thank-you notes, Christmas cards from patients, one of the VA magazines, a job recruitment letter, and one other item: a letter with my address handwritten. Even after a decade of no communication or correspondence, even through the fog of disbelief, I recognized the handwriting immediately. I managed to mute my shock and took the mail with me back to the ER. After recycling the magazine and recruitment letter, I smiled at the patients' notes, trying to recall the faces of the veterans behind the season's greetings, but it was impossible.

Then, for the rest of the shift, I contemplated what to do

with the remaining piece of mail. I couldn't read it at work, and risk losing focus. As far as I was concerned, I had forgiven my father years ago and could coast through the rest of my life father-free. It was a kind of forgiveness that happened when I wasn't paying attention, on some date and time that had passed in peaceful anonymity. Given that he was the one who had abandoned me, who had walked out of my life without giving the explanation I already knew, I had no regrets about the one-sidedness of the forgiveness. In his absence, forgiveness felt easy. It's always easier to maintain a positive vibration away from negativity than in its presence—for the same reason that it's easier to be kind on the yoga mat than while stuck in traffic. He was gone. I was free. I had dealt with it honestly. I had done the right thing—I had forgiven him. I was content that I had moved on.

Now that he had returned to my life, in whatever capacity his letter might hold, what did that mean for me and my easy forgiveness? I ran through the many possibilities for his having sent the letter. He might have been totally transformed and was reaching out now, in the ultimate expression of enlightenment. I decided quickly that that was definitely *not* the case. If that was true, he would have done more than passively sending a letter via hospital mail, which roughly approximates the delivery rate of a balloon telegraph. He was a physician himself, so he had to know that.

Maybe he was slowly dying, and as his last vestiges of vitality ebbed, he had had an unshakable awakening and was reaching out so he could finally convey his remorse.

Nah. More likely—actually, yes, definitely the case—the letter was a half-inflated test balloon released into the sky, merely a wisp of an effort to see if I might be willing to do the work, to ameliorate his feelings about his life. (That's how he had always operated, and I had never observed in him anything indicating that he would ever change his way of being in the world.) But the last thing I had time to do right now was someone else's emotional, psychological, and spiritual work—especially since I had already learned that it was impossible anyway.

I crammed the envelope into the bottom of my bag and returned to my own duties.

The letter was still in my bag, unread, when Nurse Bill knocked on the entrance to the doctors' section of the ER. "I just put in a guy with a cut on his hand. A Mr. Williams. He's a little nutty. Hopefully, you can just get him in and out fast."

"How'd it happen?" I asked.

"He said he doesn't know. He's odd. He was out, and it happened on something or other. He said he cleaned it up before coming in. Looks simple. I irrigated it and put the laceration cart at the bedside. Want an X-ray?"

"Since I don't know the mechanism of injury, we'd better get one, to screen for foreign body or bony injury. Please give a yell when he's back."

"Okay. I'll walk him up now. Lorraine will take over when he's back from X-ray."

"Coolio. Thanks."

After reading a couple more articles in *Shambhala Sun*, I

was notified that Mr. Williams was back from radiology. As I approached the room, I saw a young man pacing. He was talking to himself, at times attempting to muffle shouts as he alternated between wringing his hands and slapping his forehead with his fist. I scanned the room. No one else was with him. Nurse Lorraine was sitting in the nurses' station writing up her notes. When she saw me, she said, "We got a live one, Doc. In and out, *please*. His wound is ready."

I pulled up the X-ray on my screen and was happy to see it was normal: bones intact with good alignment, no foreign body and only minimal soft-tissue swelling in the palmar region, which was, presumably, where I'd see the laceration. With the hope that this would be a quick suture and discharge, I approached the patient's room.

I tapped at the room's entrance. "Hello, Mr. Williams."

He looked up at me, blurting, "Hi, hi, hello, ma'am. Doctor. I mean, hello, Doctor, ma'am." He glanced away and continued to pace.

Maintaining my position in the doorway, I said. "Mr. Williams, why don't you have a seat on the stretcher here while we chat?" He was clean shaven with olive skin and large hazel eyes and other features that would have made him look like a native in most parts of the world. His straight brown hair was neatly cut, but disheveled at his forehead. A blood streak on his half-untucked oxford shirt was only barely perceptible against the dark background of the navy-blue cotton material.

He lowered his head. "Yes, ma'am." He sat down, flopped

his body back on the bed, and began repeatedly crossing and uncrossing his legs. I approached the right side of the stretcher, leaving both the door and the curtain to the room open. When interviewing patients, my practice is to provide them with whatever privacy I can, but in this case, I felt it more prudent to interview Mr. Williams in full view of the rest of the department. Doctors gain this instinct with practice. Sometimes we misread, but often we do not.

Mr. Williams's chatter stopped, but he kept crossing and uncrossing his legs. Every once in a while, his entire body would jump as if he had been startled, and his eyes would dart back and forth as he squealed, "Shhhh!"

I interrupted his dialogue with himself. "Mr. Williams, I'm Dr. Harper. I don't think I said that when I first came in. I hear you have a cut on your hand. Just so you know, I looked at your X-ray and it looks normal, which is good news. What happened?"

His movements stopped for a moment. "I cut my hand a little while ago. My friend cleaned it off for me. She brought me here," he said, flinging his right hand toward my face.

"How did it happen?"

"I don't know. I don't know. I was out with my friend, and it happened. Fast. I don't know. But she cleaned it." He began to rock and rub the back of his hand. "She cleaned it. She cleaned it. She cleaned it and wrapped it up," he replied as he jumped. "Oh!" he exclaimed, then covered his mouth with his left hand.

"Are you sure you don't remember anything about how this happened? I just ask because most people remember at least something."

He looked at me but said nothing. His eyes were glassy pools of erratic terror.

"Hmmm, well, do you recall if your injuries involved a knife or a gun?" Because these are potentially reportable injuries, I always made sure to ask this when the cause of injury was unclear.

"No. No. It was fast. I don't know, I don't know. We were out. No. My friend, she told me. She brought me here. She cleaned it." He suddenly yelled, "Oh!" and then jerked his head to the side as his legs began to quiver. He ran his left hand over his head and down his neck before placing it on his chest and curling it into a fist, which he then raised to his mouth in what appeared to be horror. "No, no, it's okay. It's okay. It's okay," he muttered into his chest.

"Huh. Well, can you feel and move your fingers?"

"Yes," he responded, holding his hand in front of his face, moving each finger in wide, slow, undulating movements, before plopping his hand back on the table palm up with a thud that made both of us jump.

"Mr. Williams, are you okay?"

His attention darted back to me. "Yes. I'm okay, I'm okay. I'm okay, I'm okay," he said as he curled and uncurled his fingers into a fist, which he brushed over his mumbling lips.

"Mr. Williams, what's going on?" I asked gently.

"They're following me!" he exclaimed, covering his mouth again. He looked from side to side and then down at his chest as he began to whimper incomprehensibly.

"Who is following you?"

"They are. You can ask my sister. She called. I can call her. But she bothers me. But we can call her. I don't know."

The evaluation was becoming more complicated. My priority now had to be to address the laceration quickly so we could move on to the more pressing concerns.

"Now, Mr. Williams, the cuts on your hand are a little deep, so I recommend I put in some stitches to close them up."

"Okay, Doctor."

"Have you had stitches before?"

He shook his head.

As I set up the instruments on the bedside table, I explained the procedure. He lay back on the stretcher like a rod. It was anyone's guess what he heard between me and the voices in his head. "Now, Mr. Williams, we will begin. Again, the numbing medicine will burn at first, and then your hand will feel numb. It's very important that you stay very, very still. You can say whatever you want, just don't move, okay?"

"Okay."

"Ready?"

His left hand was balled up into a fist. He chewed on his thumb as he mumbled, "Yes," and then squeezed his eyes shut tight.

"You'll feel a pinch now." He lay there stiffly as I pierced his palm several times to deposit the anesthesia. "All done with that part." He sighed and glanced down at the V-shaped cut at the fleshy part of his palm, near the base of his thumb, which now oozed a red mixture of blood and lidocaine. Testing the area to make sure it was properly anesthetized, I inquired if he felt any pain. He indicated that he did not. As I placed the lidocaine and needle aside, he gasped again and then looked away. I loaded the suture on my needle driver before looking up to inform him that I was about to begin. But before I could, his entire body jumped. The instruments slid to the side of the tray, and the bottle of lidocaine toppled to its side and then clanked against the raised edge of the table.

He looked to the far corner of the room and yelled, "Stop it!" to whatever ghosts were there.

"Mr. Williams, are you with me?" I asked in a manner that sounded far calmer than I actually felt. I took deep breaths to still my palpitations, to cool the warmth rising in my chest. I looked through the open door to see Lorraine staring at me wide-eyed over her computer.

Mr. Williams looked back toward me. His body was still tense, and each limb was rigid on the bed, as if secured by suction cups. But his face softened, and his eyes were pleading. "Yes, yes, Doctor."

"Mr. Williams, do you still want to proceed?"

"Yes. Okay. Yes, yes."

"You just have to stay really still—perfectly still. If you move, I can't put in the sutures."

There are times when we take an uncompromising stance with patients, when we tell them to either cooperate or leave. But sometimes a softer approach is necessary. This patient seemed too fragile: I knew I would have to nurture him through the process like a doting aunt.

A third of the way through the procedure, he suddenly drew up his legs and before I could ask him to stop, he said, "It's okay, it's okay. You're okay. She's okay. We are safe here. It's okay."

I held my instruments in the air as the suture dangled between us. I waited for the outburst to pass. I waited to complete the world's fastest sutures. I thought about just stopping, even contemplated zipping through a simple continuous running suture (a type of stitch where the sutures aren't separated. You simply place throw after throw, then tie the suture material off at the end so that the tissue is connected by one long piece of suture material. The benefit of this stitch is that it prioritizes speed. The downfall is that if it breaks anywhere along the material, the entire closure comes apart), but finally reminded myself that this was his hand and I should do the sutures for the most effective wound healing, so that he would have the best chance of retaining its function. But the key was still to finish fast.

He shifted his gaze to the needle driver and forceps and then to the black nylon thread pulled taut. He then looked over to the scissors and other sharp instruments to my right. His eyes parked there, and I lowered my hands to rest my instruments on the tray. I laid the suture down so it wouldn't injure him and left the untied suture in place of the most recent stitch. I felt myself drawing my tray of sharps closer to me. He exhaled and appeared to settle again, reminding himself aloud that he was okay, I was okay, and he was safe. Within moments, I completed the fastest sutures I had ever thrown.

"All done!" I announced as I collected the instruments. I undraped his hand and asked him to wait where he was, so the nurse could clean and dress the stitched-up wound.

He lay on the stretcher, clasping and unclasping his hands, exclaiming "No!" and then slapping himself on the thighs and forehead. I reminded him not to do anything to hurt his already injured hand.

This was not going to be a quick treat-and-street. Sure, now that I'd stitched him up, I could have given him his papers and sent him on his way. This sort of thing happens all the time: We ignore the inconvenient problem because it doesn't have a rapidly accessible answer. As a physician, I cannot fix intimate partner violence, homelessness, addiction, or their brethren in one ER encounter. I can help, but I can't fix them, so it can feel easier to focus instead on what I *can* fix, the laceration I can suture shut. Asking the other questions opens a Pandora's box. Heaven forbid a patient said, "Yes, my boyfriend stabbed me; and he hits me all the time." Then I'd have to offer comforting words, followed by a call to social services—and we all know that social work involvement can prolong a patient's ER visit by several hours. But what's even worse is when I ask the question, and the patient declines assistance. Their doing so shouldn't feel like a personal affront, but for an instant, it can. Of course, if a patient declines help, that has nothing to do with me personally. Clearly, I'll go home to my life and not be beaten just the same. Perhaps what bothers me most is the raw realization that I care more deeply for the welfare of another human being than he cares for himself, and that that human being will leave my care to suffer more needless violence.

Even though I had no idea what had happened to Mr. Williams, I could see that this man was seriously ill. There was the problem of his injury, yes, but there was also a more penetrating problem of his psyche.

"Mr. Williams, you seem very upset, very anxious."

"Yes, yes."

"I think it could be a good idea for you to speak with the psychiatrist. He could help you feel less anxious. What do you think?"

"Yes, yes. He can help?"

"Absolutely. Would you also like some medicine to calm down?" He bobbed his head in compliance. "All right. Why don't we have you change into a gown and we'll check some labs just to make sure everything is okay."

"Okay, Doctor."

He was fragile but compliant. I walked over to Lorraine, relieved to be safely out of his room.

Lorraine looked up at me. "Good to go, Doc?"

I pulled my chair over to her and looked back to the room to make sure Mr. Williams was out of earshot. He was pacing again, resuming the argument with himself, one that, sadly, he appeared to be losing.

I leaned in close to Lorraine. "I cannot discharge this man. He is truly not stable. I don't have much information on him, so I can't know how close this psychosis is to his baseline. I'm very sorry, but I have to keep him on one-to-one observation because he certainly can't leave unless Psychiatry clears him. We'll need to get some labs for medical clearance, too. Let's have him get changed, the way we do with all psychiatric patients. Amazingly, he has agreed to everything. He's very redirectable and cooperative."

As I passed the triage area on my way to the psychiatric department, the triage nurse, Steve, called out to me. "Dr. Harper, can you come here a minute?"

"Yup. Are there more people out there to be seen?"

"Not exactly," he replied.

With coffee in hand, I leaned on the desk next to him, waiting for his update, but mostly I was stealing a lovely opportunity to quietly sip coffee in a department still filled with Sunday morning calm.

"There are some detectives out here waiting to talk with you."

"City police? About what?"

"Something about a murder. Apparently, that last patient—"

"You mean the only patient in the department?"

"Yeah, the patient is a suspect in a murder that happened in Old City this morning."

"Whhaaaat?!" I set my coffee down and took a seat next to Steve. "Okay, wait a second. What happened?"

"I don't know all the details, but the cops were saying an old woman was stabbed in Old City outside her church and they got a tip that led them to Mr. Williams, so they followed him here."

"How long have the cops been here?"

I looked out and saw three middle-aged men in suits sitting in a semicircle. One was leaning forward with a notepad in hand, joking with the other two, who were seated casually as if in reclining chairs.

"I dunno, maybe thirty minutes or so. But they've been on the case since the tip."

I thought back to how I had been in the room with Mr. Williams alone. I recalled him mumbling to himself and staring at the sharp instruments as I repaired his hand. I remembered the exact moment my gut told me that he and I were both unsafe there, and then the moment my instinct told me I could and must deliver us from that danger quickly. At that same moment, unbeknownst to either of us, the police were just outside, waiting for us both.

"So, you mean we were all back there with this guy who had probably just murdered someone while the cops sat outside in the waiting room joking? I was actually in the room *alone* suturing him, and none of those cops thought it a good idea to alert the staff or maybe even come back to the department to make sure we were safe?"

Steve frowned. "Yeah, that's a good point, Doc," he said. "Guess not."

I picked up my mug and headed toward the waiting room. As I approached the officers, all three stood up, each one of them at least six feet tall.

"Doc, you're taking care of Mr. Paul Williams?" one of the detectives asked. I nodded. Apparently, as they explained, my patient had been witnessed attacking an elderly woman, and the police were in the process of obtaining a warrant for his arrest.

"Is he good for us to take to the station?"

"Well, he's okay *medically*. I just had to stitch him up, and in that respect he's fine. But he is banana nuts. I mean nuts and berries not okay."

"Is that a medical term, Doc?" one of the white detectives asked, throwing his head back in laughter.

"Yes, it's one of our new terms. But in all seriousness, I've just ordered him some medication to help calm him down. In my opinion, he is truly psychotic. I'm having the psychiatrist see him."

"C'mon, Doc. Don't you think he's just faking? Pretty convenient to be mentally ill all of a sudden," the black detective said with a smirk.

I smiled because I knew that the acute onset of an assortment of medical symptoms when a person is arrested or doesn't want to report to work on a nice day are all epidemics that present to the ER. "Yeah, I have to tell you, I've seen a lot of people malingering or, as you say, faking. I've seen a lot of mentally ill people, too. Either he's ill or he's an Academy Award–winning actor, and an actor he is not. Sorry."

The detectives shuffled around. They seemed disappointed. I told them that I was still waiting for lab results, and more critically, the psychiatrist would need to see the patient before any decision could be made.

"We think it's best if some of our guys stay in the department," one of the detectives said. "We spoke to the VA police, but they don't have the staff to leave a couple of their guys here the whole time. Okay if we set up here for a while?"

"Of course. I think it's safer, too. Right now he's fine. He was redirectable all along and should be medicated now. He's honestly more cooperative than many, perhaps even more than the majority, of the sane patients I've treated," I said, smiling.

"Okay, Doc. We got you." It was nice to hear. It was the type of collegial collaboration I was used to with the police in the ER back in my South Bronx days.

I turned to Steve and called through the triage window. "Please show the detectives back. They're gonna hang out for a while. Introduce them. Make them comfortable," I said.

The psychiatrist on call was not in the psychiatric ER but undoubtedly sleeping in the on-call room. I asked the psych nurse to page him to the main ER and then walked back to the department to update the staff.

I turned to Lorraine. "I know he's calm right now, but

given everything that's occurred," I said, recalling Mr. Williams's behavior during suturing, "I think it's safer to do restraints until he's medicated. That will give us time to see that he's really psychiatrically stable and not a danger to himself or staff." I glanced over into Mr. Williams's room; he was still agitated but compliant. I saw that Mr. Carey was just being wheeled back to the room next to his.

Mr. Carey was a frequent flyer at the ER, someone who was once known to drive himself there weekly. When he arrived, he'd saunter through the waiting room and then stroll up to triage. The moment he thought he was within view, his pain would mysteriously intensify, to the point where he'd be doubled over, instantly unable to walk. He would begin shaking violently and scream in pain. Patients with gunshot wounds or kidney stones and women in labor didn't even scream like that—they were the howls of someone who was insisting on full submission to his demands. Predictably, he would begin acting out convulsions, pausing only to explain that his symptoms had been evaluated for over a year with exhaustive tests, including labs, CTs, MRIs, ultrasounds, urine tests, endoscopies, and colonoscopies, that had all, sadly—audible sniff—yielded only normal results. He would then go on to explain that, thankfully, his incapacitating pain was singularly responsive to a couple of rounds of intravenous Dilaudid.

I made sure to stand in the hallway as he rolled by, so that he could see me. He knew that I was one of the physicians

221

who would not give him narcotic medication, so it was likely he would walk out at any minute. I had seen him do it before.

"Lorraine, maybe we can just do restraints on his feet," I said, referring again to Mr. Williams. "Or perhaps feet and one arm so that he can still eat and use the urinal. Whatever you think. Just let me know."

"Okay, Doc."

I wrapped my arms tighter around myself, shivering in my fleece, trying to keep the dry, chill air of the department at bay. Mr. Carey was on my left, Mr. Williams on my right. To my left, a medically well man with no diagnoses in his medical record except for nonspecific abdominal pain and mild reflux. His room was a theater of unparalleled noise. To my right, a psychotic man in mental distress. Nurses Lorraine and Bill were both with a calm Mr. Williams to administer medications and place restraints. I saw Lorraine speaking to him, presumably explaining what was about to happen. He slowly extended his left leg for her to affix it to the stretcher. Then the right leg he granted to Bill, who tied it to the bed. Next, he extended his left arm so it could be secured. Lorraine placed a urinal within reach on his right side. Mr. Williams kept his arm perfectly still as Bill started an IV to administer the sedative Ativan and draw blood. Lorraine removed two pills from a cup and raised them to Mr. Williams's mouth. Mr. Williams lifted his chin and parted his lips to receive the meds.

I stood outside Mr. Carey's door. "Mr. Carey, abdominal pain again?"

He shrieked something with a discernible "yes" in the middle.

"Well, in that case we'll do the same workup," I responded, before returning to my desk.

"Wait, Doc! I'll need pain medicine first, before I can let you do anything!"

"Sure. I think it's safest to give you a really strong antacid medication for your gastric reflux. That should help your pain while we get your blood work and X-ray completed."

"No, I don't want that! I need pain medicine. I won't do anything without pain medicine!" he screamed, and then resumed his kicking and flailing.

I turned away from him. "You certainly have the right to refuse evaluation and any offered treatment. If you don't want those things, you will need to leave."

He continued to thrash about on the stretcher. "*I am not leaving!*" he shrieked. "I am not doing any useless tests, and I am *not* leaving!"

As I made my way back to my desk, I called out to the clerk, "Please call the hospital police to help Mr. Carey out of the department."

Lorraine called out, "Dr. Harper. Psychiatry."

I picked up the call and introduced myself.

"I'm one of the moonlighters, Ken. What's up?"

"Well, we have a murder case." I updated him about Mr. Williams and the detectives waiting for his psychiatric evaluation.

"I'll come right down. This is a little complicated legally.

Let me see the patient, then make a couple of phone calls. I'll get back to you." Ken was always very formal in his presentation. He wore white standard-fit cotton button-down shirts and plain dress shoes, and his language always matched his attire. He was also quite thorough and, despite his mechanical tone, clearly cared about doing right by his patients.

As Mr. Carey's yelling intensified with the arrival of the VA police, I felt my father's letter burning a hole in my bag—both, I knew, were best ignored so I could wrap up my work and be ready for the psychiatric input on Mr. Williams when Ken called back.

Lorraine again called out to me. "Doc, I'm sending a call in to you. It's Psych again."

"I saw Mr. Williams," Ken said. "I agree with you. He's psychotic and needs psychiatric inpatient stabilization. He can be hospitalized in a mental institution and be under arrest. It happens all the time. Unfortunately, it would be against hospital policy here to admit a person under arrest," he said, sighing heavily. "So, I'll have to write up my assessment, and then he'll be released to the police. He'll have to get his care through the prison system. It's also true that psychiatric care in the prison system is inferior. It's a shame, but it's out of our control. We'll keep him here until the police have their warrant. I spoke to the police already. Everyone's on the same page."

"Yeah, it's a shame the way our systems fail patients."

"It's all we can do."

"Thank you, Ken."

I checked the clock: fifteen minutes until the day doc was to arrive. I looked back toward Room 17 to see Mr. Williams lying still on the stretcher, his eyelids soft. His hand had been sewn, his clothing changed to psychiatric scrubs, his shoes replaced by hospital socks, his agitation soothed by Ativan and Geodon. Now he could finally rest.

The VA police I'd called for a belligerent Mr. Carey were still with him. Negotiations had resulted in the police putting on their gloves and surrounding his stretcher. Apparently, Mr. Carey was still refusing to get up and walk back to the car he had used to drive himself here. Nursing slid open the glass doors of his room as the police wheeled Mr. Carey's bed out the back entrance of the ER.

The clerk looked at the video feed of the scene outside and dissolved into laughter. "Wow, Mr. Carey just got up and gave the police the finger, and now he's walking away. What an ass!" he chuckled. "You know, he's walking just fine. Guess his pain got better!"

I packed up my things, wondering how Mr. Williams's story would be told days later in the news, weeks later in court. Would the prosecutor conjure a story of a savage, cold-blooded killer? The "If it bleeds, it leads" mentality gives a distorted sense of reality. Mr. Williams was no more ferocious than the kids who pretend to look tough on Instagram, or the commercial artist from the burbs who raps about the hard life in the hood that he never had. But this sensationalism sells images that, while disconnected from the truth, can have very real consequences.

I thought about how such portrayals separated us from our human inclination to empathize and forgive. What had happened was horrific on every level, but news reports in cases like these often circumvent the root issues. Instead, they typically skim the surface to sell fear, to stoke animosity. It was tragic that Mr. Williams had attacked that woman. Sad that her heart had stopped when her lung collapsed around it. Sad that she was murdered by a stranger when all she had wanted to do was go to church. It was also sad that this tormented man was caught between this reality and the world of his mind. I couldn't know what had brought him to that point. I did know that most psychotic people aren't violent; in fact, it's the sane ones who pose the greatest physical threat to others and commit the most violence. I knew that Mr. Williams had once been functional enough to be enlisted in the armed services. Then something had happened. Perhaps he had a genetic predisposition that timed a late-onset schizophrenic break. But this is rare. Usually, there is trauma that triggers a psychic separation. And usually this trauma is layered onto prior unresolved traumas to tip the balance to an altered state. As the spirit struggles for protection, it can become frozen, can splinter, shatter, quiver inside not knowing how to heal.

I could only imagine the trauma caused to the woman's family as well as to the larger community by her murder. Her killing was as heartrending as it was unjust. It was also true that Mr. Williams's suffering was so great that he had experienced a break. Of course, as is the case in adulthood, his trauma is his own responsibility. His actions are his to bear. But the trauma of every veteran and, more broadly, every person, is also ours. I couldn't say for sure, but most likely Mr. Williams, as in the case of the many veterans whose mug shots we see on the news or who sleep invisibly under bridges, had been broken by the combat he waged in our name. So, his trauma was ours, too—our trauma, our pain, our responsibility. Just more evidence of the interconnectedness of all beings.

The arrival of the day team signaled the end of my shift. On my way to the parking lot, I searched my phone for the song "Rosebush Inside." This would be a fitting soundtrack for my trip home. The guitar strummed as I pulled out of the hospital lot. The day before, I had listened to a podcast on NPR about Moreese Bickham. In 1958, two local police in Louisiana who were reportedly also Ku Klux Klansmen made good on their promise to exact revenge for an argument in a bar and came to Bickham's home in the middle of the night armed with guns. In this attempted murder, one shot Mr. Bickham in the stomach. In self-defense, Mr. Bickham returned fire, striking and killing both men. An all-white Louisiana jury sentenced Mr. Bickham to death. In 1996, after he'd spent thirty-seven and a half years in prison, the governor commuted his sentence, and at the age of seventy-eight he was released. While incarcerated, Mr. Bickham had made it his mission to be of service. He became a minister and a mentor to other inmates. He also found refuge in a rose garden. Of his cherished roses, he said to an interviewer who visited him in prison before his release, "I want to introduce you to the beautiful rosebush . . . This one here is my favorite. I named it after my wife, Ernestine—a beautiful pink rose. And some way or another, I keep it trimmed and uniform looking, too. I call it my beauty. I know it sounds funny, but these are my company keepers. I enjoy these bushes. See, if it wasn't for these bushes, I wouldn't have nothing to do. So, these bushes have come to be close, close, very close to me."

After his release, Mr. Bickham said he bore no anger toward anyone. Instead, he practiced gratitude for his many blessings. I imagine it was so that the society that had robbed him of his physical autonomy could not also steal his peace of mind. For the rest of his life he continued to hold the system accountable through his work advocating against the death penalty. To me, he was someone who learned to live without bitterness and who savored every ray of freedom. In this way, he harbored unconditional love that few ever choose to achieve.

I pulled into the parking lot and began the walk across the street to my condo. Like the lull of the night shift, the quiet time of being home was rife with things to contemplate. Forgiveness had freed Moreese Bickham when his body was enslaved. While suturing up Mr. Williams, I had allowed myself to be guided by a deep forgiveness for his erratic behavior, which might have escalated to danger, and this had likely saved my life. Then, of course, the fact he hadn't harmed me may have saved his life, too.

It's the same calculation we make when we physically take down an agitated patient in the ER. There are risks and benefits to both the action and the inaction, so the critical question *before* either is chosen is whether action is truly necessary. So, too, the calculation taken regarding when and how we expose our military men and women to danger: We have taken too many liberties with their health. They are put in too many situations that should have never occurred in the first place. When danger is unavoidable, they deserve to be well supported during and then after the trauma they experience. We failed Mr. Williams the way we failed Ms. Honor. In the same way Vicki found healing in forgiveness, we as a nation need to do so as well. We need to acknowledge our errors openly, earn the forgiveness for the failures, and, most important, do better from that place of loving-kindness.

Forgiveness condones nothing, but it does cast off the chains of anger, judgment, resentment, denial, and pain that choke growth. In this way, it allows for life, for freedom. So that's what's at stake when it comes to forgiveness: freedom. With this freedom we can feel better, be better, and choose better next time.

Now that everything I had known had fallen away, I knew I would have to sit in this space of transition. Despite the end of relationships with my ex-husband and then ex-partner, followed by the end of what I thought the practice of medicine was and would be, I had decided to stay in Philadelphia for the time being. I had put down roots here. I had achieved my goal of becoming a doctor. I had been married—and then divorced because I had grown up. I had purchased a condo in Center City, which I had filled with paintings from contemporary artists for inspiration and with incense, candles, chants, and totems of "oms" for balance. And I had feasted on pure love. I had never *needed* Colin. Real love never needs. Part of pure love is knowing when to stay, when to yield, when to hunker down, and, ultimately, whether it's after an hour, a decade, or the duration of this brief life, when to go.

I was in a new phase, one in which I realized that simply continuing to accomplish more of those goals that the mainstream world deemed important—in my career, in my personal life—would only lead to the desire for more and more to feed an insatiable hunger. This, too, would require forgiveness.

As I entered my apartment, I recalled the letter from my father, still lying at the bottom of my bag. I was calm now. For the first time in my life, I was dedicated to self-care in an unrepentant way. I was dedicated to loving myself so fully that the natural response was also to love unconditionally any authenticity I found in others. In this, too, was the freedom of knowing that another person's journey had little to do with my own. Forgiveness was a natural response, the only one that really mattered. It meant that I could be okay with the possibility, indeed, the likelihood, that my father had reached out to me selfishly, and that was the best he could or chose to do. I was okay, too, with deferring my response.

I pulled the letter out of the bag. It occurred to me, too,

that there was a possibility that the correspondence could be some version of a sincere explanation. I took out a fresh envelope, then stamped and addressed it so I could mail him my updated contact information should he want to speak to me. Putting the envelope aside, I opened his letter.

Inside was a Christmas card containing a piece of white paper folded into quarters. I carefully unfolded it and proceeded to read a handwritten note from a man lamenting his life. He expressed that he had finally taken responsibility for everything he had done. He went on to share that since he had broken off all contact with me, he had tried to learn about my life through periodic online searches about what I was doing, where I was living, who I had become. He congratulated me on the awards I'd received for patient care and compassionate doctoring he'd come across.

The letter ended with his phone number in the event that one day I might be open to speaking with him. Before I realized what I was doing, my hands were rifling through my bag for my cell phone. Seconds later there was ringing. At the third ring it dawned upon me that I hadn't planned what I would say.

Then I heard, "Hello?"

"Hello, it's Michele Harper," I said.

There was a pause followed quickly by, "Michele, I am so happy to hear from you. How *are* you?" I felt my father's voice cracking on the other side of the line.

We spoke cordially in a cursory way. I caught him up on what I was doing—that I was an emergency room doctor at the VA hospital in Philadelphia—and plans for the future. He repeated much of the letter's content, then updated me: He was still living in the suburbs of rural Pennsylvania, still practicing medicine, mostly in the prison system.

Then he surprised me. "Michele, I've always remembered what you told me in one of our last conversations. You said to me, 'You don't *own anything*.' And you were right. I've remembered those words so many times through the years. It wasn't until I *owned* all of my mistakes—and that was so painful—that I could begin to change. I've dedicated myself to getting better over the last twenty years."

My jaw dropped and my heart melted to discover that he had heard anything I said all those years ago.

"That's fantastic," I said. "What a wonderful transformation for you!"

While it was too early to gauge the extent of his growth, I had never expected even this revelation from him. While it wasn't exactly an apology, it was an important admission. As far as I was concerned, no matter what happened next, a miraculous metamorphosis had already occurred.

He asked if we could meet next month, and I agreed. He would travel to Philadelphia and stay in a hotel. In a few minutes, we exchanged good-byes and the call was over.

Relief washed over me. I fell into the familiar warmth I experienced in yoga and meditation. With that one conversation, my father had given me a gift of an explanation decades in the making.

I recalled Heidi Bourne's piece on *Mettā* and forgiveness.

Yes, I was still me, but I had evolved over the years. Perhaps he was still himself, but maybe different, too. I realized in the moment that whether he had or hadn't changed mattered far less to me than the fact that I truly had forgiven him. I condoned nothing about the way he had lived. My appreciation of the exchange was in no way contingent on the fantasy that he was entirely or even partially reformed; nor had our conversation meant he was welcome back in my life. *But* I was proud of the fact that my forgiveness of the childhood I didn't have, my forgiveness of never having the father I wanted or deserved, my forgiveness of his brokenness was real. In this forgiving, I had allowed us both to heal. So, Heidi was right, "No big deal. And yet, it was everything."

TEN

Sitting with Olivia

———— ————

I SAT, craving stillness and knowing there was no other way to it than to let the craving go, to allow it to pass. I thought of a quote by Thich Nhat Hanh, the renowned spiritual leader and peace activist: "Letting go gives us freedom, and freedom is the only condition for happiness. If, in our heart, we still cling to anything—anger, anxiety, or possessions—we cannot be free." So, I sat there, waiting, trying not to grip too hard. After the last line of the chant, the vibration of "om namah shivaya" lingered in the meditation center. The center's being a fifteen-minute walk from my home made it possible for me to attend sessions once or twice each week. The walk itself served as part of the ritual.

I heard the shuffle of the monk's assistant as he turned off the music, which indicated it was time for silent meditation. The last echo of the prayer radiated through each of my cells from my core out through the tips of my fingers and toes, taking with it the globs of tension, the clumps of resistance shaken loose by the reverberation. In its wake, emptiness. The crown of my head floated upward. My hands poised featherlight on my thighs.

Yes, this is it, that longed-for nugget of thoughtlessness.

With that, a stream of thoughts flooded my mind. What would I do about my current job? What would be my next big career move—no, *life* move? What would I do when Colin returned? Should I hear him out? More important, how would I forgive him for the immense pain I had allowed him to cause both of us?

Doh! I had done it again. Here I was, sitting next to myself, realizing again that judgment in the meditation space opens the gates for more judgment, more assessment, more momentum in confusing directions. Just like in yoga, injury comes easily when we slide into common ego patterns of pushing for a certain pose, a certain shape, a certain look on the surface. In the same way, emotional harm comes easily when we push from habit without directed intention.

As my chest tightened, I watched my thoughts, like quicksand, settle on my body. My palms became hot, and my skin felt compressed. The collar of my sweater was suddenly itchy, and just as suddenly, I couldn't change position because of the intractable discomfort in my lower back. These were my cues to stop. Stop caring about my sweater, about the sore spot that had popped up on my right ankle— wait, had I just been bitten by a mosquito?

No. Just. Stop.

A thought bubble titled "Job" appeared in my consciousness. I saw myself sitting cross-legged as the bubble drifted by. My arms didn't move, my mind didn't shift. My ribs expanded and contracted with every breath as "Job" dissipated. My body melted into a velvety warmth. Everything fell away. A soft black sheet of space enveloped me. A watery ebony diffused into waves of crimson, auburn, yellow, and gold. I drifted in the middle, stable, secure, grounded, yoked to nothing. There I met a buoyant clarity as vibrant blue light radiated from my throat, opening as a luminous, expanding orb. A shiver ran down my upper back. A vision of Colin appeared. In his face, sincerity; in his eyes, love. I was filled with warmth, yet I was attached to nothing. The blue pulsated with each heartbeat, expanding and contracting with the rhythm of my breath. At my core was a dark magma from which emanated a knowing. It was less a voice, more a whisper. Not words, but a message whose translation contained in it the Ho'oponopono prayer:

I love you. Breathe in. I'm sorry. Breathe out. Please forgive me. Breathe in. Thank you. Breathe out. I loved you. Breathe in. I'm sorry. Breathe out. Please forgive me. Breathe in. Thank you. Breathe out. I release you. I loved you. I've released you. I release you. I release you.

The image and the voice dissolved into the radiating indigo that kept me upright, rooted, steady, firm, easy. Then, nothing.

The blue orb was swallowed back into the black pulsation that smoothed to gray. As I floated in stillness, the meditation bell rang. My bare feet on the ground felt chilly from the fall evening. I wrapped my wool sweater more snugly across my chest and scratched that itchy patch on my neck. My shoulders hung weightless at my sides. My throat was open.

I gathered my things and got ready to leave. I decided to keep my phone off. It was time to gently process what had happened. I had been meditating on my own for a while, but my practice remained sporadic. In this time of transition, I knew I needed some structure as I rededicated myself to the new life path I was crafting, and these Thursday evening sessions had been a helpful tool.

As I left the center, crisp air brushed my face. The storefront lights on Pine Street appeared more radiant. The cityscape was a collage of colors: robust greens, soothing browns, lustrous yellows. For the first time in a long time, I was awash in freedom. For the first time, perhaps ever, I was truly comfortable. I knew that after letting go, there is forgiveness; after forgiveness, there is faith. My key now was a radical alignment with truth, a radical faith that in leaning into love and letting go of everything else, the path unfolds as it should. I walked home amid leaves sailing to the ground—a gentle landing from a life cycle well spent.

When I opened the door to my condo, sweet spicy air filled my lungs. Yes, this was why I always burned incense: for that instant of remembering the moment I returned home.

The next morning, my phone alarm tore me from sleep.

My first thought was that I must set a gentler alert. My eyes peeled open. Well, my right eye did, but my left was submerged deep in my pillow. As soon as I opened my eyes, I felt a quick tightening in my chest: the familiar anxiety. I stopped and let myself appreciate the warm embrace of the covers and the glow of my meditation message from the day before. The habitual grip of fear melted as one pattern gave way to the next. This new pattern was allowing me to feel supported, because life is better when I allow myself to feel that way. This morning I was appreciative of how the sky-blue throw that swaddled my face felt like a handful of dandelion seeds. I emerged from bed still feeling light from my night of meditation, my yoga of letting go.

Twenty-four minutes later—I have the time from my front door to the front gate of the hospital down to a science, provided there is no traffic—I approached the hospital entrance and waved a blind "hello" to the officer, whom I couldn't possibly recognize in the darkness. With my coffee in hand, I checked the sign-outs from the night before. All were straightforward.

Like clockwork, the new patients started to arrive: three nonurgent patients for the fast-track area of the ER flashed on the board, followed by four patients for the main ER. One patient was quickly tracked to Room 12. The comments listed "HTN, headache." Another tracked to Room 7: "alcohol detox, depression." Knowing I would need to see the hypertensive patient first, I checked the triage and vitals for the detox patient. They were normal for this forty-year-old man, with the exception of mild tachycardia, an elevated heart rate. He looked stable and medically healthy. The triage nurse, Angela, came over to give the roll call.

"Mornin', Dr. Harper, the bus has arrived! I just brought back two because of acuity. A hypertensive lady with a headache. Here're her vitals and EKG," she said, passing me the first of two. "I already put in her labs. I know you like a chest X-ray, so I ordered that, too. Do you still want it?"

"Yes, please. Can you add a head CT, no contrast, so we can look into that headache? I'll see her first, I just want to get her into the CT queue since they've had a long wait. I'll cancel it if I change my mind."

"Will do. There's also a guy with depression, Mr. Wade, here for detox. Here's his EKG," she said, handing me the second electrocardiogram. "Said he'd been drinking on his way here. You'll see his heart rate is a little tachy, at one-nineteen, but he's fine."

I quickly entered the standard orders for psychiatric clearance and alcohol intoxication for Mr. Wade, complete with a banana bag (an IV solution comprising normal saline and vitamins. The yellow color of the fluid is the reason for the nickname), before starting on my hypertensive patient.

Two additional main ER patients awaited triage. At 8:55 a.m., I heard the thunderous greeting of my co-attending for the day. Dale was always punctual. He arrived early and then worked slowly. He, too, had a love of coffee, and I always enjoyed his political commentary and music selections for the shift. Even if it was a busy day, it was fun to have him by my side.

"Hello, dear," he bellowed.

"Lovely to see you, sir. Such a peaceful morning, and now you've arrived with the bus."

"Yeah, well, what's new? It's always busy here anymore. I knew you were gonna be here, so I brought an additional container of my extra-dark-roast coffee with a hint of coconut oil. It's magic in a cup! I know we talked about coconut oil losing its superfood status with that questionable cholesterol information, but I figure in moderation, it's a justifiable indulgence."

I adored Dale's coffee: There was something special about that added coconut nectar. His kindness in bringing this gift so we could enjoy it together during a busy shift made our morning ritual that much more delicious.

"To the elixir of life," he cheered as he handed me a thermos filled with my portion of coffee and then raised the other in a gesture for us to toast.

"Thank you again, Dale. I'll be right back after I see this lady with a hypertensive urgency situation."

I double-checked her electronic medical record: Olivia Hernandez, fifty-seven-year-old female with a history of hypertension, anemia, reflux, and being overweight. Her only medication was HCTZ, for her blood pressure. No allergies. Her medical record showed she had regular medical follow-ups and was pretty healthy. All appeared unremarkable.

I approached the room to see a woman who would have appeared much younger than her stated age if not for the mask of fatigue heavy on her face. She was neatly dressed in a pressed white dress shirt, snug blue slacks, and black ballet flats. Her thick black hair was secured in a casual ponytail that fell limp over her shoulder. While she was listed as over-weight, it couldn't have been by more than fifteen pounds or so. She was arranging her phone so that it lay visible on her lap and had placed her black satchel next to her on the stretcher when I approached her room.

"Good morning, Ms. Hernandez. I'm Dr. Harper. And how are you today?"

"Good morning, Doctor. I'm good, good. I called to see my doctor this morning because I haven't been feeling well. I just knew my blood pressure was up." She paused. "Well, I should be more specific." Her phone beeped, and she silenced it before putting it away. "I'm sorry, Doctor," she said, letting out a long exhalation and rubbing her forehead. "Where was I? Yes, I called my doctor because I've been getting these headaches sometimes. When I saw the nurse, my blood pressure was high, one-eighty over one-ten, so she said I had to come to the ER to be seen because it was too high for the clinic."

"Of course, Ms. Hernandez. That makes sense," I said, smiling at her. "How are you feeling now?"

"Actually, right now, I feel good. When I came to the hospital, I had a terrible headache. It was pressure all over here," she stated, motioning across her forehead to both temples. She gave me a puzzled look. "Huh, you know my headache is still there, but better. I'm sorry, I feel so silly. I feel fine now." She seemed embarrassed as she turned to look at the monitor behind her. "How's my blood pressure now? I'm so sorry to take up your time here. I should go," she said, as she started to gather her belongings.

"Let's see," I said, walking over to the monitor. "Let me ask you a couple more questions while it's checking." I hit the button to cycle the blood pressure. "So, I know you said you feel fine now. Did you have any chest pain, heart racing, or difficulty breathing?" She shook her head, indicating that she did not. "Any change in vision, numbness, weakness, leg swelling?" Again, no. "Difficulty urinating, blood in urine."

"No."

"And now the headache is mild?"

"Yes. Now that I'm here, I'm fine. My goodness. I'm so sorry to waste everyone's time!"

"This is no waste of time." I looked up at the monitor to see the new reading. "And your blood pressure is coming down a little since you came in. Now it's one-sixty-nine over ninety-eight."

"Still high, but better. Thank goodness!"

"It is. And we haven't done a thing to you." We both chuckled. "Any recent change in your medications?"

"No, Doctor. I'm only on one medication anyway. It's called hydro . . . hydry-something."

"Yes, your hydrochlorothiazide."

"That's it. I take it every day like clockwork."

"Hmmm. Any smoking, drinking, drugs?"

"Goodness no. I mean, maybe a glass of wine rarely, but I really don't even do that. Trust me, I'm sure I need a drink, but these days I really can't." She laughed, a moment of levity.

"What about stress?"

She let out a sigh. "Geez," she said, slicking back the sides of her ponytail. "Do I have stress!"

I paused, squinting at her. "You seem like you're a caretaker. What's going on with your stress?"

"Well, Doc, as I sit here, my husband is also at the hospital. I'm sorry. That's why I was checking my phone earlier. He was recently diagnosed with cancer. Unfortunately, it's already spread. He's been in and out of the hospital, back and forth to doctors' appointments. And then we . . . well, now *I* also take care of my granddaughter. She's four and autistic. Her parents . . ." She stopped and shook her head. "Well, anyway, we have full custody of her now. I just haven't had the time for anything."

"Of course. That makes a lot of sense."

"I haven't been eating as well as I used to," she said, pulling at her blouse and then pointing to the buttons anchoring the fabric gaping open over her belly. "Doctor, this just happened last month." She rolled her eyes upward as if scanning for glimpses of her former self.

"Well, you certainly do have a lot that you're juggling right now. While there are many reasons for hypertension, I'm pretty confident your recent spikes in blood pressure have a lot to do with your stress."

"I'm sure, too."

"I know you have a lot going on, but is there anything you can do to cope with the stress you're under now in some beneficial, positive ways?"

She laughed at this question. "Actually, there are some good things. My brother told me today that he can help out with appointments and errands for my husband. So, that helps."

"What about your granddaughter?"

"Yes. Her parents are my greatest disappointment. They weren't doing anything for her, so we've been playing catch-up. I'm pretty sure we'll qualify for some kind of services for her, but I have to look into it. So much legal work. Let's not discuss that right now, Doctor, if you want my blood pressure to stay down!"

"I gotcha," I said, smiling. "So, the good news is that it sounds like there are some possibilities of assistance that will free up time and space for you to take care of *yourself*."

"Take care of *myself*," she said dreamily. "I'd like to get back to that. I *need* to."

"Are there things that you enjoy? Some kind of physical activity, for example, could help with your blood pressure, mindfulness, and general wellness."

"Believe it or not, I used to do martial arts. I did it for years. I really enjoyed it. There was something very calming about it, too. My sensei was a spiritual man, so he emphasized meditation in our practice. Because of him, I started meditating on my own. Just five or ten minutes a day. It really helped. I've been wanting to get back to it."

"That's something that could really help you now. Even as you finagle your schedule, you might just start the meditation again."

"That's true."

"So, here's the thing: I have a feeling that your blood pressure elevation and headaches are stress-related. Now, I don't want you to think I'm minimizing the importance of your high blood pressure by saying that. But we know there's a powerful mind-body connection. Stress can lead to heart attack, stress can lead to stroke, stress can lead to infection. You get the idea. Because of this, even when I feel your symptoms are due to stress, we should check your blood to take a look at your kidneys, do a chest X-ray to take a look at your heart and lungs, and an EKG as well to look at your heart. Let's do a head CT, too, to make sure there's no bleeding or other abnormality, given your new headaches in the setting of elevated blood pressure. This may seem like overkill, since I'm pretty confident they'll all be normal, but I still think we should check to be safe. Make sense?"

"It does. I have a feeling they will all be normal, too. I think it's just stress. I don't want to take up any more of your time. But since I'm already here, I might as well get checked out, because goodness only knows when I can come back. You're right. I definitely can't afford to get sick now, so better to play it safe."

I nodded. "And you could even practice that meditation you mentioned while we're waiting for your results."

Ms. Hernandez reclined on the stretcher, and her face softened into a smile. "Good idea."

"Excellent. Just relax. Do you want the lights on or off?"

"Off is good. Thank you."

I flipped the light switch and as I left the room, I heard Transportation calling to take Ms. Hernandez up to radiology. Perfect timing. After refreshing my computer screen, I saw that all her labs, as expected, were normal.

Next, I moved on to Abraham Wade, a tall, muscular white man who'd come in for alcohol detox and depression; his repeat vitals were normal. I tapped on the door and completed the routine introductions. His hair looked as if it had been recently cut, and it was dark and slick with the same sweat that ringed his collar. Although he had told Angela he'd just been drinking, he appeared sober. He didn't seem to have any acute medical issues. He explained that after being in the military, he had had a bout of prescription drug abuse: He'd been prescribed oxycodone for the chronic back pain he developed during his deployment overseas. His mental health care notes explained that his primary care provider and pain management specialists had worked together to get him on a non-narcotic pain regimen. When I asked him about this, Mr. Wade agreed that it was partially true, but added that it was truer to say that he had simply decided he didn't want to be addicted to narcotics anymore.

He had stopped taking them and started working out more, which had alleviated his pain.

I completed the required history and exam and then prepared to get back to my coconut coffee.

"Well, Mr. Wade, my part is done. I just do the medical screening. Your labs are all cooking, and I'm pretty confident they'll be fine. The other parts, the depression and alcohol use, you and the psychiatrist will discuss," I stated as I began to back out of the room.

"Doctor, do you know who the psychiatrist is? Do you think he'll send me home? I mean, I'm not suicidal or nuthin'. I was just so desperate. I want to live. I want to be better. I'm a good guy," he said, pointing at his chest. "I'm *really* a good guy. You might not know that from all the shitty things I've done, but I am."

"I believe you. We all do shitty things sometimes," I said, unable to stifle some knowing laughter.

"Yeah, right?" he said, nodding.

"As for who's on, it's Dr. Masetti. I really don't want to speak for him. He's super nice and thoughtful. A really sweet man. I know he will do whatever he can for you. Anything else before I go?"

"Ma'am, I just really want to do this," he continued. "It's time. I never talked about my drinking when I was here before," he pleaded as he kneaded his hands.

I took a couple of steps toward him and rested against the sink to show that I was listening.

"Ever since I got out, I've been drinking. Come to think of it, I was drinking before the military. I remember I would drink when I was a kid. When my father wasn't home, which was always—thank God, because he was a tyrant—I would break into the liquor cabinet and take a bottle out for me and my friends. I did stop drinking when I enlisted. I mean I only drank between deployments. I liked to say that I would only have a drink with dinner or socially." He frowned and wrung his hands. "But I was pretty social, Doc." He laughed. "Come to think of it, ma'am, I was always a mess. Ever since I was little, I tensed up when men yelled. So, what do I do? I join the military, of all places," he said, throwing up his hands. "When I got back, I was always wound up. I'd start sweating in crowds—markets, malls. God forbid a car would backfire. I didn't even realize until recently that that is *not* normal." He paused. "I'd just go home and have a drink.

"Ma'am, I had a good job. I was the foreman at a big construction company and ran my own side business, too, doing floors, some painting. I was doing great. But then I started drinking more and more. I didn't know what was happening. I mean, I literally didn't know because I would black out. My business was the first to go. Then my wife left with my son, just last month. She did the right thing, too, Doctor. I was an asshole." He paused, frowning again. "Look, I'm sorry. I know you don't have time for all this. I know you have other patients."

I was listening to him, taking it all in. "It's okay. I have a minute before I have to scoot."

"Thank you, ma'am. I just wanted to ask," he said, clearing his throat. "Well, I'm sorry. I mean, first, do you even know how I ended up here? A couple weeks ago I somehow called my wife—or ex-wife; I don't even know what she is now, but I called her. I don't know what happened. I was drunk. She had left to stay with her parents and stopped taking my calls the week before, so she didn't even get my voice mail until the morning. She checked it and heard me spewing craziness. She tried calling me at home; I didn't answer. She called work, but they said I wasn't there. She was too afraid to come home, and I don't blame her.

"I woke up to men in SWAT gear breaking down my door. Meanwhile, I'm curled up in a fetal position on the floor with my guns laid out around me. Next thing I knew, all these armed men rushed the room. They got a call from my ex saying she had to flee the house the month before because her husband, who's ex-military, is a depressed alcoholic and he just left a message screaming about how he's gonna kill himself. To tell you the truth about it, I was really embarrassed, but I was also more than a little pissed off that they busted my doors. The police took me to the closest ER, but I refused treatment. Instead, I went home to fix my fucking doors."

Realizing he'd used an expletive, he interjected, "Oh, I'm sorry, Doctor. Please excuse my language."

He continued: "Yesterday I blacked out and woke up this afternoon with my bedroom door on the floor—I don't think I ever fixed it right. Two empty bottles of vodka were on the floor from I don't know where. I had a voice mail from work, since I was a no-show, and one from my five-year-old son, who I haven't seen in three weeks. So today, I drove myself in. There really isn't much left for me to lose. I *have* to do this. I know this isn't your decision, but I just want everyone to know. I want everyone to know now that I need help. I'm a good guy under all this bullshit. Oh, sorry again for that."

I studied his ruddy face. I felt the determination in his voice. "No worries, I get it," I said. "You're a good guy, and you'll get through this. You *are* getting through this. I'll let the psychiatrist know what we spoke about." What I meant but couldn't say to Mr. Wade, for fear of implying a promise that was not mine to make, was that I would beg Dr. Masetti to admit him to the hospital today.

"Ma'am, again, I'm sorry to keep you. I just wanted to ask you something before I went off on that long tangent. I want to ask you how hard will this be? How hard is detox?" His tone seemed to convey even more sincerity than before. He was a strong man, a smart man, one who right now was desperate and open. In this moment, he was a man who wanted with every fiber of his being to transcend this part of his life.

I looked at him, wanting that transcendence for him, too, wanting it with every fiber of my being. "That, my friend, is a good question. I'm going to tell you the truth because I think you want it, I think you deserve it, and it will only help you get through this so you can live the life you want, which is the life you deserve."

He nodded silently, listening raptly.

"Let's talk about the physical part first. It's true the body can become dependent on alcohol. Some people have more of a physical dependency than others. As you detox, you might feel anxious, you might feel sweaty. You might feel your heart racing. In severe cases, people hallucinate—and the list goes on. *But* we have medication for all that. Honestly, even if you have a seizure, heaven forbid, it's going to be okay because we can manage the physical part for you while you're here. This medicine will soothe you and help prevent any of the dangerous complications.

"That will be the easy part. Compared to what invariably follows, this will be the sweet phase of the process. The next phase will be bitter and prolonged; even unpalatable to the point of insufferable when you're back at home.

"It's the other parts," I continued, "the mental, emotional, and spiritual parts, that are harder because these are the parts that *you* have to do. Not only do you have to begin this healing while you're here, but you now have to accomplish it without the old crutch of the alcohol. Sure, alcohol can ruin your life in the long run, but it served the purpose of being a pretty powerful coping mechanism for a very long time. It was an aid that helped you survive. Now you take the alcohol away and you deal with your life sober. All that stuff that was drowned out by the alcohol when you were little, before you went to war, when you went to war, when you came back from war—now you face that stuff without the drink. We are here to help, but even with the therapists, social workers, groups, and medications, it will be challenging—but worth it. You're a strong man, and you'll get beyond this to be stronger than you've ever been, stronger than most people will ever be in their entire lives. You'll get beyond this so you can be happy, so you can have a job that fulfills you, so you can be the father you want to be to your son, so you can tell the story of your survival and your victory. This is the story that will save your life and the lives of many others, so it is truly all well worth it. And you'll need to remember this end goal every hour of every day because this will likely be the hardest thing you've ever done in your life. And you *can* do this."

He drew a deep breath and nodded as he clasped his hands in front of him. He sat upright on the bed, sturdy, preparing himself to win an exacting victory.

"Again, many good people are here to help you," I continued, "but the most important thing is that you must want this for yourself and that *you* are willing to do the work to claim it. That's the *only* way it happens. This decision to own your life every second, which will turn into every minute, which will turn into every hour, and then into each day, one day at a time. Eventually it'll be second nature. And one day soon, it won't be hard anymore. It'll just be everyday life, like breathing."

I could see the resolve in his eyes, the move he was making in allegiance to his health.

"Thank you, Doctor. Thank you."

I extended my hand. "Mr. Wade, one day come back and tell me your stories. Tell me your stories of how good it is. Just remember: First it will be challenging, and then you'll be free."

We shook hands. I felt his heartbeat pulsing in my hand. He nodded again. "Thank you. I will."

All of Ms. Hernandez's results were back. When I returned to her room, I saw her lying on the stretcher with her head resting back and her eyes closed. I knocked on the door, and she opened her eyes with a smile.

"Welcome back. All good news. Let me just cycle your blood pressure while I give you the update." I pushed the button to start the measurement again. "As we anticipated, your blood work was all normal—your kidneys, electrolytes, et cetera. Your chest X-ray was normal, and your head CT, too." The blood pressure cuff stopped cycling, and I regarded the reading. "*And*," I stated in the way of all great game show hosts, "your blood pressure is down to one-fifty over eighty-seven!"

She sighed and raised her hands in a little happy dance. "Praise Jesus. Doctor, you know I just sat here and breathed. I meditated like I used to do in martial arts. And it worked!"

It had worked. It worked better than the pill we could have given her, better than the medication we could have pushed into her veins. Sure, it's always faster in the moment to silence the body's ailments pharmacologically, to write a script in lieu of having a conversation. When your main goal is to get through each patient encounter as quickly as possible, these approaches will do. But if the goal is patient autonomy, to support patients in achieving long-term self-generated health, it's better to pay careful and thoughtful attention to the roots of what makes us healthy.

"Of course, follow up with your doctor for a blood pressure check. Best to call them today to arrange it, since they referred you to the ER today. It's still a little high, so they may need to tweak your medication. I know you're super busy and you have so much to do for your family, but your body and spirit are calling out to you, asking you to take care of yourself so you can remain the healthy, strong, caring person you are. Know what I mean?"

"I do, I do," she said, smiling.

"And that's all you need from us today. This was the universe's way of tricking you to come in simply so you could be reminded. That's it, that's your message."

As she collected her belongings and prepared to leave, Ms. Hernandez expressed her rejuvenated commitment to self-care.

"I'll write up your discharge papers so you can get on with your life. Any questions?"

"None at all. Thank you, Doctor."

I signed my notes for Mr. Wade and then completed discharge papers for Ms. Hernandez. Dale had picked up the two new patients. Five new patients were in fast-track, and it looked like the three patients in the waiting room who had just signed in would be coming over to the main ER—two medical and one psych. Perfect timing, because both Dale and I were just tucking in the patients before them.

As I waited for the new patients to be triaged, I considered the journeys of Mr. Wade and Ms. Hernandez. Mr. Wade's door to healing had opened in a loud and dramatic way: by armed men who had literally come knocking at his door (before breaking it down). He had been passed out on the floor, a limp heap of a man, and then he had been jolted awake. Ms. Hernandez's call came quietly—a slow throb at her temples, a dull ache of fatigue that goaded her to get checked out "just in case." As she was waiting for the results of our tests, she had brought herself to stillness; she had found a way to gather herself into a healing peace.

Both these patients had let go in their own ways as they moved toward health. And isn't that how healing usually happens? In these ordinary times, in these everyday moments, people open themselves to what serves them most.

It's with these chronic states of *dis*-ease that prescriptions of traditional medicine fall short. Don't get me wrong— heaven forbid, if I'm hit by a car or contract bacterial meningitis, 911 me to the nearest ER for the best that traditional medicine has got. (And, yes, vaccinations are good.) But once traditional medicine has delivered me from that acute phase of illness, I know that if I want to stay well, the root and core of that health come only from complementary means. It was acupuncture that alleviated my seasonal allergies, thereby permitting me to stop an exhausting regimen of allergy shots, nasal sprays, eye drops, and two different antihistamine pills. It is yoga, cardio, and Pilates that keep my body limber and strong. Maintaining a healthy diet—well, that does everything. My meditation practice has made it possible for me to live in a way that is nourishing while the rest falls away. For the chronic conditions of daily life, it is these other modalities that will stave off depression, anxiety, hypertension, high cholesterol, diabetes, obesity, heart disease, stroke, and cancers so that we can find a better quality of life than we can by adding yet another bottle of pills.

Ms. Hernandez, Mr. Wade, and patients like them inspire me. I, too, knew instinctively to stop fighting for my life and begin *allowing* it. In this way, I had to let my attachment to Colin float away in order to permit both of us to be our best selves. He needed time and space to decide whether he would be a warrior in this life. My decision had been made: I was a warrior already. Whether it took Colin the seventy years it had taken my father or simply the next twenty, he deserved to go at his own pace, as I deserved to continue at mine. With that realization, I had walked away from Colin softly, quietly, and decidedly. Somehow, with only the effort it takes to let go, receive, and believe, what my heart called for would come in. My *dis*-ease would dissolve. This time now was the invitation to be okay, even happy, without filling in the details of how my love would come to me, how my family would look, or what the final destination of my professional journey would be. While I figured out the next bold career move, I would continue to serve. This was the time to live my love now. No better time.

ELEVEN

Jenny and Mary:
What Falls Away

MY FIRST DAY BACK, and I can't stop thinking about the goo I discovered between the pages of the in-flight magazine.

Come to think of it, I'm probably one of the few people in the world who actually reads the in-flight magazine tucked in the seat pocket in front of us when we fly. Maybe it's an extension of my type-A personality, but part of me believes there could be some critical morsel of information in it. Or it could be that I'm still gullible enough to think that if the airline put it there, it must contain a safety update necessary for my survival or, at the very least, a surprise deal on the afternoon snack. Or maybe I'll be tipped off about the perfect place for Sunday night jazz in Nashville, should I ever go there. For all these reasons, one of the first things I do whenever I board a plane is check out the magazine. And after years of my being vigilant, my last trip delivered.

In the midst of everything—the job switches, the blockage of my complementary medicine center, the breakup with Colin, the what-the-hell-am-I-doing-with-my-life internal conversations—I had forgotten that I had volunteered to attend the VA conference on women's health. While it turned out to be, arguably and quite sadly, one of the poorest-quality conferences I had ever attended in my medical career in terms of providing the attendees with comprehensive, up-to-date medical information, there were a couple of highlights: The patient models who coached us in optimizing our physical exam skills were masterful, and a female veteran gave a heartfelt talk about how she had survived her time in the military. While I was used to providing female veterans with general medical care and treating their military wounds related to sexual assault and harassment, there were other aggressions on military women I hadn't yet considered before hearing this vet share her experience: for example, the various chronic pain syndromes that developed from their being forced to use gear that had been specifically designed for male bodies. While women were allowed in the military, in most cases they weren't permitted to exist on an equal footing with men.

There were three nonclinical elements that made the conference worthwhile as well. My fellow conference participants were delightful. Of course, we swapped the all-too-familiar stories of the creative workaround strategies we used to compensate for the lack of resources at our respective sites, from the Carolinas to Colorado. The fact that this was often done over quesadillas and drinks by the pool only added to the camaraderie. Hearing about the dedication of my colleagues in other parts of the country was a nice reminder that there are still doctors and nurses out there who aren't willing to give up on the art of medicine or on the people who rely upon it.

Then there was the hotel fitness center's steam room, the discovery of which inspired an unreasonable amount of joy in me. I can always find refuge in a steam room. Whenever I use one, any toxic thoughts expire on the vapor, leaving space for positive inspiration. Assuming a sense of ease as I breathe in the sweltering steam is the only way the extreme heat becomes tolerable. This requires the engagement of every component of yoga—the body, the breath, and the mind. In this way, within seconds of my entering its quarters, the steam room challenges me to achieve alignment. My reward? An ultimate fast track to the infinite.

As if primed by the steam, I was now ready for the pièce de résistance of the trip. On my flight back to Philadelphia, after I collapsed into my window seat, I picked up the inflight magazine. After skimming the ads for watches and suitcases, followed by hot new restaurant listings across the globe, I happened upon an article about the life cycle of butterflies. As I learned in my youth from *The Very Hungry Caterpillar*, a butterfly begins in the caterpillar stage, in which it eats and eats and eats, and finally ends up majestically bewinged. But I didn't know that after this growing caterpillar enters its cocoon for the pupal stage, it literally turns into goo. Apparently, scientists don't understand why or how the caterpillar form breaks down during this period of transformation in order to emerge as a butterfly.

As I placed the magazine back into the seat pocket, a thought struck me: That's truly how it is, isn't it? As long as we're willing to move forward, to nourish our body and spirit and allow for the disintegration of any attachment to patterns that do not serve us, without our understanding exactly how the next bits will fall into place, beautiful outcomes do unfold.

Back at work, I continued to ponder this process of transformation. Breaking my butterfly daydreams, an announcement blared over the speaker system: *Campus response parking lot level C. Campus response parking lot level C.* Within minutes, the campus response team, the group of men and women designated to respond to potential medical emergencies throughout the hospital, were rolling in a stretcher bearing a small, limp patient: a child. A distressed young man followed quickly behind them. The team assembled in Room 4, encircling the child. I stood at the foot of the bed and supervised Jaya, the medicine resident on her ER rotation, as she assisted in care for the patient.

"What's going on?" Jaya asked the team leader.

"Twenty-two-month-old with febrile seizure. She was here today with her dad, visiting one of the patients. She has no past medical history. Dad said she's had a cold for the past couple days and fever this morning. She started to have jerking movements in the parking lot, and a bystander called for help. She has appeared post-ictal the whole time with us. Dad said the seizure lasted for less than a minute, and she's been like this since. No seizure activity with us."

The child was small and beautiful in her golden yellow dress decorated with unicorns. Soft brown curls swayed from side to side as she stirred languidly on the bed. Her thick black eyelashes fluttered as we positioned her on our stretcher. Her eyelids stayed closed, then tensed for a moment as if she were warding off a nightmare, before relaxing back to whatever dream state she was in. The nurses rapidly scrambled for pediatric supplies to get a set of vitals. When we hooked her up to the monitor, we found her heart rate was in the 120s, saturating 97 percent on room air. Her temperature was 100.5, and her blood sugar was a reassuring 89.

"Jaya, please go talk to Dad and get any additional history and come back with the scoop," I instructed. "We'll continue the case together at that time."

I turned to the tech. "Liza, please help completely undress baby Jenny. We need full exposure."

To the nurse assigned to Room 4, I said, "Ted, we'll need basic labs, chest X-ray, and urine. Let's also give a bolus of normal saline at ten cc/kg."

Jaya returned, and we examined this little doll together. She moved her extremities spontaneously in reaction to our gentle touch. She flinched, and her lips curled in a slow-motion cry, when the IV was inserted, and then two tears formed in her right eye before she slipped back into her stupor. While she wasn't yet alert, at least she was intermittently responsive. Her skin was flawless from the crown of her head to the bottom of her itty-bitty toes. Her diaper was normal and wet with clear, light yellow urine. Jaya lifted the child's eyelids to reveal large green eyes with pupils that reacted to light. Tympanic membranes and oropharynx normal. Lungs clear and heart sounds normal. The abdomen was soft and appeared to be non-tender.

"Jaya, you want me to enter those orders for you?" I asked.

"Please, Dr. Harper."

At the computer, I clicked on all the boxes I needed: chemistry, CBC, urine, chest X-ray, liver function tests. Wait, I said to myself, I wasn't going to order liver function tests. There honestly was no reason to get LFTs in a healthy, febrile seizure patient. But this child wasn't waking up, so the situation could be turning into a more serious medical issue. I moved the cursor over the LFTs to unclick it, but then I didn't. I couldn't bring my index finger to press the button down.

Something just felt wrong. I had no good reason to suspect badness here; after all, apart from her semiconscious state, the child had a normal exam.

The dad, who was now at the patient's bedside after we had completed our initial evaluation, appeared to be appropriately concerned as he caressed the child lovingly between medical interventions. The stories he'd given to the rapid-response team and to Jaya were consistent, but I decided to go ahead with the test anyway. There were greater crimes than adding one extra, non-evidence-based test to a pediatric patient's evaluation. Perhaps there was some metabolic issue that LFTs would help elucidate, I said to myself, knowing full well that this was untrue. I signed my orders and waited.

"Dr. Harper, we might as well get this kid ready for transfer. Even if it turns out to be a simple seizure in the end, she's not waking up, so she needs to go to a pediatric hospital for further testing and observation," Jaya said.

"One hundred percent agreed, Jaya. And this is why you're one of my favorites." I smiled.

"So far, we know her exam, vitals, blood sugar, and urinalysis are negative. Her chemistry is fine, too. Her X-rays are pending. I'll call the Children's Hospital now for transfer," Jaya said.

As Jaya went to do that, Dr. Berry, the attending working the fast-track section of the ER, approached her to see if she would be interested in helping with the reduction of an acutely dislocated shoulder when we finished our case. I told Jaya I'd finish the calls and paperwork on our case so she could complete the joint reduction with Dr. Berry.

Minutes later, when Jenny's X-rays came in, I looked at them. Pediatric films can be challenging because a child's bones are immature, but nothing acute jumped out at me: clear lungs that were well inflated with no pneumonia, fluid, or pneumothorax. Her CBC and chemistry were unremarkable. The patient had been accepted to the nearest children's hospital, which was conveniently less than a mile away. The hospital was sending its ambulance unit to pick her up. Seconds later, EMS bundled the child back onto the gurney to leave. I clicked back into her chart and saw that her LFTs had just come back: They were five and six times the normal limits. Just as I registered concern, I got a call from radiology.

"Hello, Dr. Wechsler of Radiology here. Do you have the child just X-rayed for febrile seizure?"

"Yes, baby Jenny."

"Okay. No source of infection here, the heart and lungs look good, but there are fractures. Looks like different stages of healing. Mostly old and well healed. Possibly one or two newer ones, I can't say that for sure, but I can say this is not good."

I looked back to see the gurney rolling out of the department, the father following close behind, his face twisted in fright, his knit hat clenched in his fist and drawn close to his quivering lips as he asked the paramedics if his baby would be okay. Her mother had arrived and was being comforted by an older woman who appeared to be either her mother or his. The family trailed out behind the gurney of the child who was broken by one if not all of them.

"Thank you, Dr. Wechsler. This is bad, very bad. I'd better call Children's Hospital to update them before the patient arrives."

I called the accepting physician, whom I had spoken to just minutes earlier. "Dr. Pierre, Dr. Harper again. I want to give you a terrible update. The child is on her way over to you. Just as EMS rolled her out the door, I got these last two pieces of information. Her LFTs are significantly elevated, and she has multiple rib fractures on X-ray. I'm really concerned this child's altered mental status is the result of blunt trauma, probably liver injury from blunt trauma as well, which explains why the LFTs are through the roof. She certainly needs a trauma workup. I'm sorry."

It was possible the child had some critical metabolic issue that had led to liver failure and recurrent seizures. It was possible those fractures were from those same seizures and had gone undiagnosed. Yes, that was all possible, and there are case presentations written on this very phenomenon. There are also times when your gut tells you otherwise, when you're in the presence of another body and can't help but feel its energy and hear the whisper of its silenced story. This limp, semiconscious child had been beaten—beaten to convulsion, beaten to fracture, beaten to a bleeding liver.

"Got it" was Dr. Pierre's response. The accepting doc at the other end of a transfer call never says much. The case isn't real until it arrives. The information isn't true until it's verified. Right now, my call to her was only adding to her workload, so "got it" was a reasonable response. Plus, we ER docs stand witness to human suffering too frequently. It was draining and depressing, and often left us with only enough hope to muster those two words.

So, days later, when the update came that the father had been charged with abuse, that he had caused the retinal hemorrhages, cerebral contusion, multiple fractures, and liver laceration, we couldn't say we were surprised. It wasn't because he "fit the part," whatever that means. My snapshot of him in the middle of the ER hadn't fit any particular stereotype. No, we weren't surprised because this is what we do. I imagine every forensic examiner has the same reaction. It's horrifying and sad when you realize something terrible about another human being, yes. But—and this is a disturbing commentary on humanity—it can no longer be called surprising. It wasn't yet known if the mother, who had stood by for the past twenty-two months as he abused their daughter, would also be charged: The calculation as to what extent the "bystander" is complicit, it seems to me, is always complicated and often tortured.

As I ended the call with Dr. Pierre, Nurse Carrenza approached me.

"EMS just rolled in a respiratory arrest that they intubated in the field from a nursing home. Only the rotating dental resident is in there now, so we could really use you."

"Of course," I said as I followed her to Room 20.

As I entered the room, one paramedic was bagging the patient and a tech was doing chest compressions. One nurse was placing the patient on a monitor, and another was obtaining a second IV; EMS had already placed one.

"Hello, all. I'm Dr. Harper. What's the story?"

"Hey, Doc. Ms. Mary Giannetta is a seventy-eight-year-old woman with diabetes and a heart condition," one of the paramedics explained. "She was in distress at the nursing home. Actually, her family found her and alerted the staff. Did the nursing home call for notification?"

We all shook our heads.

"Geez. Of course not." The paramedic sighed. "When we arrived, she was barely breathing, and then lost what thready pulse she had. PEA on monitor. Unknown down-time. She's been with us about fifteen minutes and has had three rounds of epi. The last dose was given approximately one minute ago. Accu-Chek two-fifty. We put a twenty-gauge in her right AC and obviously intubated in the field."

"Thank you. Y'all did everything," I said as I walked over to Ms. Giannetta's right side. "Now that she's on our monitor, can we hold CPR to get a pulse check and switch roles so EMS can be on their way? Respiratory, please hold bagging, too, while I listen to the chest. No breathing, no breath sounds." I placed my second and third fingers on the patient's carotid artery while watching the monitor. "No pulse." One slow line snaked across the screen with mild variations. "PEA. Please resume CPR with compressions, bagging, and let's give an epi."

I looked over at Crystal, the nurse who was recording for the code, and asked her to please advise me at two-minute intervals so we could keep track of our pulse and rhythm checks as well as when medication administration would be due. Over that time, I completed my physical exam: Good air entry in both lungs, and the patient's oxygen saturations were in the high nineties, with the respiratory therapist's continuous bagging, both signs pointing to the endotracheal tube being in good position. The patient's fine salt-and-pepper hair bounced with each chest compression. Her plump olive skin was segmented by deep laugh lines, giving her face a wise and honest cast. Her heavy lids were coated with shimmery peach eye shadow and charcoal eyeliner; I lifted them to reveal large black pupils that were fixed and dilated. Her body showed no signs of trauma and no signs of movement save for the give-and-take of CPR. Her belly was soft.

"Four minutes. It's time for epi this time," Crystal announced.

No pulse at the neck. No pulse at the groin. The same fine line slithered across the screen, but this time it was almost entirely flat.

"Another epi, please, and let's resume. Can someone go get the ultrasound for the next check? She's down at least nineteen minutes, with no return of circulation and no meaningful rhythm. If people don't disagree, I think we should call it at the next check unless there's a change."

"Definitely," Crystal said. Heads nodded all around.

"Is anyone here with her?" I asked.

Tina, the tech, responded. "No. EMS said the family stayed behind because they had to make some phone calls. They should be arriving soon."

"Okay," I said.

We heard a clanking, crunching sound.

"There goes a rib!" said Jared, the nurse who was performing compressions.

"Yeah, but what's the clanking?" Crystal asked.

We looked around the room. The bed was locked, and

no equipment had fallen. Tina, the tech on the left side of the bed, lifted Ms. Giannetta's left arm, raising her hand. Her nails were painted with frosted pearl polish. On her ring finger: a two-toned wedding band of yellow and white gold curled around three tiny antique diamonds whose settings resembled a row of gilded baby's breath buds. Her fingers curled limply over Tina's palm.

Tina looked up at us. "Her ring. Her wedding band is hitting the bars." She then lowered Ms. Giannetta's arm gently to the bed and positioned it closer to her body. No more rattle.

"Time!" Crystal said again.

No pulse. No heart sounds. No breath sounds. An increasingly fine and slow slither across the monitor that was now arguably flat by all measurements.

"Nuthin', guys," I said and pulled over the ultrasound machine. "Let me just check her heart for any beating." I squirted a quick blob of jelly over the center of her chest and then placed the probe on her anterior chest wall, over the region of her heart. Turning my gaze to the screen of the ultrasound machine, I saw the thick gray chambers of the heart lying flat, with stagnant black holes for blood. The only movement was my hand swiping back and forth as I viewed the still, silent organ.

I removed the probe and replaced it in its holster. Looking up at the clock, I announced, "Time of death, four twenty-nine p.m." I continued: "Okay, I'll get to the documentation and calls to the medical examiner and organ donation. Can y'all please tell me if and when the family arrives."

"Sure thing," Crystal replied.

I sat at my desk, asked the clerk to get the medical examiner on the phone, and opened my chart to document the code.

"Doc . . . Doc?" A voice called out in hesitant upspeak.

I turned to see Crystal with one foot in Ms. Giannetta's room and another pointed toward me.

"Yeah?" I said.

She was looking at me quizzically, her mouth open, but instead of words, she let out a sigh.

"Ummmm." She narrowed her eyes and pursed her lips. "You know, I think you should just come back here and see."

I felt a kind of instant dread. You never want to hear one of your colleagues say, "I think you should take another look at this." Just as you never want to look down to see that the ultrasound-guided peripheral IV it took you four attempts and twenty minutes to place has red blood pulsing up into the IV tubing.

After two deep breaths, I followed Crystal back into the room.

Tina looked up at me with wide eyes as Crystal closed the curtain behind me. "Doc, she's breathing!"

"What are you talking about?" I asked.

Tina pointed. "Doc, look."

Condensation and slow swooshes of air rose and fell in

the endotracheal tube. I listened at the patient's chest to confirm. The monitor still showed a flatline. No pulses at the carotid. No pulsation at the femoral.

"Crystal, can you come over here and check, too?" I asked.

Crystal walked slowly to the left of the bed and placed the pads of her index and middle fingers to the neck. "Nothing," she reported. Then she shifted to the left groin. "Wow . . . nothing." She shook her head in disbelief.

We looked at each other.

I frowned and crossed my arms. "I've never seen anything like this."

"Doc, I'm a heck of a lot older than you, and *I've* never, ever seen this happen. I mean, what the heck?!"

"Jackie!" I called out to the clerk. "Please tell the medical examiner never mind." I looked back at Crystal. "I guess we have to cancel that time of death stuff and continue the code. While the ACLS algorithm doesn't specify a case like this, I'm pretty positive I can't pronounce someone dead who is still breathing. How she's all of a sudden breathing while still having no cardiac activity, I have no idea."

Crystal went back to the code sheet to document this new turn of events and called the crew back in.

"Jackie, please call Dr. DeLaurentis, since he's covering the ICU. Luckily, he also happens to be her cardiologist. I'll have to run this by him, I guess, for the sake of completeness. Can you also please call Respiratory to hook her up to a ventilator and page for portable chest X-Ray to confirm the endotracheal tube placement while we sort all this out? Crystal, she has two good peripheral IVs, so let's start dopamine in one, since there's clearly no blood pressure. Peripheral access is good enough for now, since I don't know how far we can go with this."

"Sure. Uh, I guess we kinda have to, don't we?" Crystal said.

My medical training was little help in explaining what Ms. Giannetta was experiencing. Not only was this not the stuff of medical science, but it demonstrated its limitations in comprehending life on this plane.

"Dr. Harper, Dr. DeLaurentis on the phone," Jackie called out.

I picked up my phone and relayed the whole fantastic story to him. He was a kind, gentle doctor, and I imagined that was why he received the story much better than I would have if someone had called me out of the blue to assume care of a patient who was, technically, not really alive.

I hung up and told the team: "Dr. DeLaurentis will be right down, and he's gonna call the family, too. He knows them well."

Within moments, Dr. DeLaurentis appeared in the ER. One never recalls exactly the details of an exchange with Dr. DeLaurentis because he swoops in mesmerizing. After the interaction with DeLaurentis, you know you've seen a man approaching in a smart Italian suit with coordinating classic leather dress shoes and belt, there's the black hair combed back with a slight wave, and then the smile that illuminates the whole ER with its sincerity. But then the details of the conversation become hazy; you simply recall that he was there, and that made everything better. He approached me with outstretched arms.

"I don't know what to say. I mean, when you called, I believed you, but I didn't really *believe* you. I just examined her, and *what*?"

"I know!"

"Well, let me have a talk with the family, since I know them and I'd be the one to admit her. I'll take it from here and let you know how it goes."

"Please let me know if you need anything."

It was always a lovefest with the debonair Dr. DeLaurentis. Later, after the family had arrived and he'd spoken to them, I had just finished repairing a leg laceration in Room 6 when he pulled up a chair next to mine.

"I had a long talk with the family. I was honest with them. I told them that given how long she's been down with her heart not beating, there's no way she'd have any meaningful brain function if, on the slim chance, she were to survive. They all said this is not what she would have wanted; she wanted to go peacefully and with dignity when it was her time. We turned off the vent and the dopamine. They're sitting with her now. They're just waiting for one of the daughters-in-law to arrive. Do you mind if we use your room for a little while longer? If this goes on too long, I promise we'll move upstairs."

"Not a problem. Please keep me posted."

"Will do," he responded before returning to the room with Ms. Giannetta's family.

I saw a woman in tears being escorted by the triage nurse to the room only several steps behind Dr. DeLaurentis. This must be the family member they had been waiting for. I saw Dr. DeLaurentis open the curtain for her and then close it. After a moment, the beeps of the monitor stopped. Soon after, Dr. DeLaurentis returned.

"She passed away. Stopped breathing."

"Just like that?" I asked.

"Just like that. Thank you for your room. The family is collecting their belongings and should be out soon. They're calling a funeral home for arrangements. You can let your nurses know they can take the body down to the morgue. Of course, since she was admitted to me, I'll call the ME and Organ Donation. She's my patient anyway, so I'll do the death certificate." He patted me on the shoulder, smiled, and left to go back to the ICU.

I walked over to the counter to get the pen I'd left there and stood writing my follow-up notes on patients. In truth, I wanted to get a glimpse of Ms. Giannetta's room. I counted three, possibly four generations around her. Then her family came out in pairs—toddlers clinging to parents and aunts, middle-aged couples, elderly adults who appeared to be siblings. Tina and Crystal removed the monitor and folded the sheet gently around Ms. Giannetta's arms. I marveled at how she had waited, how she had known. I marveled at how she hadn't left until all her family had arrived. How she had returned to say her last good-byes and only then had taken her final rest.

I felt a tap on my shoulder that made me jump.

"Oh, sorry, Doc. Just me."

It was Al, one of the custodial staff employees. He'd always check in with me about his health goals. He'd lost weight, which had allowed him to wean himself off most of his medications for high blood pressure and diabetes. I was happy to cheerlead him along from the sidelines.

He smiled, opening his arms. I leaned in to return his hug.

"What's going on?" he said. "You look spooked. How's your day going?"

"Where to begin, Al? Where to begin?" I laughed.

Should I start with the little girl who had been beaten unconscious by her father? How would I tell him that her silenced body had called out to be heard, cared for, saved? I wondered if I should go into detail about how the body can house a million truths that may not be readily apparent on the surface, or how so much wisdom flows beneath the skin. Or should I begin with the old woman who had returned from death to say her final good-byes to her family? How would I tell him that her body had been ready and at peace, but that there had been one final task for her spirit to complete before she transitioned? Should I explain that nothing in my medical books or in "science" could explain that when she was dead, she came back just long enough to wait for her loved ones to gather by her side?

Or maybe I should start by telling Al that this had been a most painful year—or rather, series of years. Should I tell him that it was probably exactly because the challenges I'd faced had taken me to the brink of despair that I had been able to uncover a newfound freedom? Should I explain that my body was punching out a message to my heart and soul, that I had learned to tap into the message again and again between shifts and heart tugs, trying to translate, but that I hadn't yet fully grasped the dialect? Should I add that I felt it had to be a message to love more no matter what, to be happy now no matter what?

Or maybe I could start by telling him that I was finally figuring out that all bodies ache with a wisdom that wants to be appreciated. And that if I were still enough to listen, if I were brave enough to be vulnerable and courageous enough to have faith in the potential of this life, I would see that I was already healed.

Baby girl Jenny would, in all likelihood, wake up to be reborn. Ms. Giannetta had had her resurrection as well. I, too, felt as if I had lived and died and lived again in the span of this one shift.

What I managed to say was "Al, this has been a crazy day in a crazy, crazy decade."

"You okay?" he asked with genuine concern.

"I'm good. And I will be better, too."

"You're gonna leave us, aren't you?"

I smiled at him, both not wanting to disappoint and not wanting to lie. "No, Al, not right now. I mean, I hope to come up with other ways to serve, other ways to be a healer, but patient care is a part of that goal, too."

"You know, Doc, folks here come and go. The good ones are pushed out, and the bad ones get promoted. I hope you stay. What you said about healing—that's why we need you here. You care about healing."

With that, I took the deepest, most warming breath of the day and then let it go, fully refreshed.

"Thank you, Al. You don't even know."

I gave his arm a squeeze before leaving to pack up my coffee cup, water bottle, and bag. I would figure it out. I'd finish out the rest of this night, this week, this month, and then this year strong, all the while listening for what I needed to hear. I remembered something I had read—*truth is that which never changes*—and it occurred to me that that eliminated most things. In my commitment to loving *true* things deeply, I had let everything else fall away in its own time and in its own way. I made a plan to wake up and practice yoga from this space of integrity tomorrow morning, whatever yoga or tomorrow might bring.

"Night, Al!"

"Good night, Doc!"

Epilogue

---

*There can be no rebirth without a dark night
of the soul, a total annihilation of all that you
believed in and thought that you were.*

—HAZRAT INAYAT KHAN

BROKENNESS CAN BE A remarkable gift. If we allow it, it can expand our space to transform—this potential space that is slight, humble, and unassuming. It may seem counterintuitive to claim the benefits of having been broken, but it is precisely when cracks appear in the bedrock of what we thought we knew that the gravity of what has fallen away becomes evident. When that bedrock is blown up by illness, a death, a breakup, a breakdown of any kind, we get the chance to look beyond the rubble to see a whole new way of life. The landscape that had been previously obscured by the towers of what we thought we knew for sure is suddenly revealed, showing us the limitations of the way things used to be.

Of course, many of us choose to live and die with that very space uncharted. Like Mr. Spano, I, too, have been so fed up with what felt like indomitable desolation that I just sifted through the wreckage and then shouldered it, dragging it along behind me, bent over by the weight of sorrow. But this devastation is a crossroads with a choice: to remain in the ashes or to forge ahead unburdened. Here is the chance to molt into a new nakedness, strengthened by the legacy of resilience to climb over the debris toward a different life.

Jeremiah wept blood into my hands in the same way that Erik's entrails wrenched him to truth. Days before baby Jenny lost her innocence to the brutality of her parents, Vicki reclaimed her freedom by rebirthing herself past cycles of abuse into a new, healthy world of her choosing. When the stories of my relationships, personal life, and career path were stripped away, I finally got to what was real: True happiness only and *always* comes from within. In these and countless other ways, there is no gain without loss. Then—there it is! First in the descent and then in the emergence from this dark night of the soul lies true integration. True caring, indeed, true living, comes from being able to hold peace and love for oneself, and from sharing that unwavering, unconditional love, knowing that all life depends on this.

This is why I choose to stand with Mary and Dominic at the threshold. Medicine, like yoga, like the entirety of this existence on earth, is a daily practice. It is the opportunity, should we choose it, to heal the human body and spirit. By healing ourselves, we heal each other. By healing each other, we heal ourselves.

This is my practice. These are my stories.

So, this is not a book about a romance or a chronicle of

loss. It is a story of love rebuilt better; the story of a butterfly birthed from goo; the story of newly grown wings that beat to a higher vibration to soar in a place of unconditional love because the truest part of me has always known and just now understands that *this* is where healing happens and *this* is where healers abide.

ACKNOWLEDGMENTS

Loving gratitude to Mom, Eileen, John, Eli (Button), Jax, Kim, and to other family—those by birth and those by selection. Thank you to those both named and unnamed in this manuscript for contributing to my evolution on the path. Thank you to my first editor, August, who helped light the fire. Thank you to Anne for being my editor, consultant, overall literary whisperer, and friend. Thank you to my literary agent, Elizabeth, who gave me the chance because she believed. Thank you to my Riverhead editor, Jake, who pushed me out of my comfort zone and into continued growth—by the way, even your dadly input was greatly appreciated. Thank you to the copy editors, for providing me with the final beatdown; after all, isn't that how ninjas are made? Thank you to Riverhead, who made the wish come true. Thank you to every spiritual teacher who kept me sane when I was pretty sure that sanity was no longer an option. And, of course, thank you to the ground that relentlessly rises up to meet us as long as we're willing to take the next step.

WORKS CITED

Bourne, H. "No Big Deal: On Metta and Forgiveness." *Lion's Roar*, July 6, 2015. https://www.lionsroar.com/no-big-deal-metta-forgiveness/.

CDC. "The Tuskegee Timeline." U.S. Public Health Service Syphilis Study at Tuskegee. Centers for Disease Control and Prevention. Atlanta, GA, December 30, 2013.

Gacki-Smith, J., et al. "Violence Against Nurses Working in US Emergency Departments." *Journal of Nursing Administration* 39, no. 7–8 (2009): 340–49.

Gindi, R., et al. "Emergency Room Use Among Adults Aged 18–64: Early Release of Estimates from the National Health Interview Survey, January–June 2011." National Center for Health Statistics. Centers for Disease Control, May 2012. https://www.cdc.gov/nchs/data/nhis/earlyrelease/emergency _room_use_january-june_2011.pdf.

Gladwell, Malcolm. *David and Goliath: Underdogs, Misfits, and the Art of Battling Giants*. New York: Little, Brown and Company, 2013.

Goodell, S., et al. "Emergency Department Utilization and Capacity." The Synthesis Project. Robert Wood Johnson Foundation. July 1, 2009. https://www.rwjf.org/en/library/research/2009/07/emergency-depart ment-utilization-and-capacity0.html.

Janocha, J., and R. Smith. "Workplace Safety and Health in the Health Care and Social Assistance Industry 2003–07." Bureau of Labor Statistics. U.S. Department of Labor, Washington, DC, August 30, 2010.

https://www.bls.gov/opub/mlr/cwc/workplace-safety-and-health-in-the
-health-care-and-social-assistance-industry-2003-07.pdf.

National Public Radio. "Rosebush Inside." *Snap Judgment*. NPR, December 1, 2014.

Reiter, Keramet. "Experimentation on Prisoners: Persistent Dilemmas in Rights and Regulations." *California Law Review* 97, no. 2 (2009): 501–66.

Sack, K. "After 37 Years in Prison, Inmate Tastes Freedom." *New York Times*, January 11, 1996.

Smith, M. "The Murder of Emmett Till." *American Experience*. PBS, 2003.

Tolle, Eckhart. *A New Earth. Awakening to Your Life's Purpose*. New York: Dutton/Penguin, 2005.

Washington, H. *Medical Apartheid: The Dark History of Medical Experimentation on Black Americans from Colonial Times to the Present*. New York: Anchor Books, 2006.